BACK TO HEALTH AMERICA

Exposing the Exploitation of American Health and Wellness

JAMES IGANI

J. Cohen Walker, Ed.

Copyright 2015

Back To Health America
by James Igani

FIRST EDITION

Printed in the United States of America

ISBN 978-0-9837229-6-0

The views and opinions expressed in this book are the sole expression and opinion of the author, which is based on the personal and practical experience of the author on the matters contained within this book and does not necessarily reflect the opinion, position or views of Foresight Book Publishing Inc., which do not endorse or warranty any claims expressed by the author or contained within this book.

All rights reserved. This book is protected by the copyright laws of the United States of America. This book may not be copied or reprinted for commercial gain or profit. Permission will be granted upon request. No part of this book may be reproduced without written permission, except for brief quotations in books and critical reviews. For information, write Foresight Book Publishing, 2101 Chestnut Street, Chattanooga, TN 37408.

FORESIGHT BOOK PUBLISHING
ForesightPublishingNow.com

Table of Contents

Disclaimer

The content of this book is provided for informational purposes only. It is not intended to be a substitute for advice from a truly qualified, competent, and unbiased physician or healthcare provider. Do not use any information contained in this text to self-diagnose, treat diseases, or prescribe or discontinue medication. If you have or suspect you have a medical condition, you are urged to contact your healthcare provider immediately. This text is intended to present a learning awareness based on my empirical knowledge gathered from years of experience, observations, research, measurement, and my own views. Those views and opinions are based solely on studies and experiments with humans in all stages of life cycle, from newborns to the elderly of different ethnicities, socioeconomic, and educational backgrounds.

I have always maintained a strong sense of skepticism, so I set out to learn about health and wellness rather than just believe and follow the views and recommendations of certain individuals, regardless of their academic degrees and/or status they have in the community. Science is knowledge; unquestioning belief in what someone else knows is ignorance. The information herein can be incorporated into a process to help you and/or your healthcare provider make informed decisions regarding dietary lifestyle choices.

My wish is that you will utilize the information I have presented to become a more productive and dependable individual, parent, family member, employee, and citizen. As I have witnessed time and time again in the lives of many of my friends, family members, and former and current patients, regardless of socioeconomic status, academic and religious background, our society has a tendency to marginalize not only those of advanced age, but those of failing health.

Dedication

I dedicate this book to my daughter and son, Shereen and Javid. Thank you for being very supportive and, on occasion, tolerating my teachings. I love you very much and without you I probably would not have the drive and urgency to be in near-perfect health. I don't want you to ever worry or be concerned about my well-being. I promise to always make the best lifestyle decisions so I have the opportunity to take care of you when you are old and frail.

Javid and Shereen, I hope you will continue to follow my wellness and disease prevention recommendations to escape unnecessary suffering from chronic degenerative diseases, be able to achieve your goals in life, be pleasantly prosperous, pass that prosperity to those you choose to love—your children and grandchildren—and spare me the greatest pain in life. Many times I have seen my patients lose their children to lifestyle diseases. I cannot fathom a greater pain than the death of a child.

The greatest gift anyone can leave behind for their children is the knowledge of attaining near-perfect health. Without it, all goals in life lose their priority and the opportunity for a do-over is shattered. This is especially true if your life ends in your mid-60s. Death is the easiest part of life. It's the other part—the suffering, loss and death of the functions, one body part at a time—that is unconscionable.

Acknowledgements

There are many people who made this book possible and it is imperative that I offer my heartfelt thanks for their support, contributions, and of course their love.

My mother, who gave me the gift of compassion, and my father, who placed great emphasis on education and sound health habits.

My friends Joann and Ken Pritchett of Cleveland, Tennessee, who inspired and helped me with the creation of my Back Safety and Wellness program in 1998.

The few supportive and encouraging members of the nursing staff at Erlanger Medical Center, Mrs. Delores McCarty's support and encouragement, and the few residents at Creekside at Shallowford Retirement Complex in Chattanooga, Tennessee, specifically Josephine Johnston, Jean Kuhnert, and the late May Streiter, for believing in me and my passion.

I extend my sincere gratitude to Patti Rievley Wagner, my children's grandmother, who gave up her home for over a year, following my nearly 15 months of homelessness, so I could fulfill my obligations as a dad during my bitter divorce.

The staff at Memorial Credit Union. Unlike most conventional banks, MCU provided much-needed financial assistance and opportunity when I was sleeping at my office or in my car. Their "Trust Based Banking" philosophy enabled me to get back on my feet and better care for my children.

I wish to thank Mr. Terry Ramey, his wife Linda, and his wonderful and friendly staff at Linda's Produce in East Ridge, Tennessee, for their excellent produce, customer service, and their kindness and generosity. Several years ago Terry offered me the privilege of purchasing their produce at his location at discounted prices. This enabled me to provide more fruits and vegetables to my family, friends, and patients so I could introduce them to healthier foods and satisfy my own insatiable appetite for produce, especially watermelons and apples.

I also wish to thank Mrs. Donna Alper who has been very instrumental and supportive. She has inspired me to finally finish writing *Back To Health America*, which was started eight years ago. Donna improved her health by following my recommendations as have many others in the past. She realized the importance of passing on this information to the unsuspecting and often suffering public so they could choose to start and enjoy their own journeys to wellness. Without her support and persistence I would have probably sat on this book for another seven years.

Finally, I wish to thank the teaching hospital's human resources staff, registered dietitians, physicians, physical therapists, and nurses with whom I worked, including their efforts to try to discredit and disparage me and my work with clients, and to almost criminalize my wellness philosophy. It was this level of ignorance and hostility along with their irresponsible behavior that made me even more determined to research and experiment to improve my own health and the health of my eager and enthusiastic clients.

Introduction

I have been called an "extremist" or "rigid" numerous times because of my plantarian lifestyle, or I've been told it's very difficult to follow and/or maintain. However, I don't see how a dietary lifestyle that's geared toward achieving wellness could or should be considered extreme. Five percent of my diet comes from junk. After all, I am a human being and every once in a while I would like to experience only five percent of what the rest of the population experiences on a daily basis. Of course I draw the line when it concerns consumption of animals and animal by-product. I am an animal lover, but above all, I love, value and protect my own body and health. The following are some extreme conditions that often crop up when my "extreme" dietary lifestyle isn't followed and maintained:

1. Strokes—losing control of half of your body, the inability to walk safely, speak clearly or swallow effectively due to a blood clot or a hemorrhage in the brain. Too many CVA (Cerebral Vascular Accident) victims live for many years with those limitations until they expire, and most are in their early 50s or 60s. This is the age bracket when we should begin to enjoy our lives.

2. Diabetes—losing a limb or two, losing eye sight, lack of sensation in the hands or feet, and captivity to routine trips to a dialysis clinic due to the effects of diabetes. Many victims seem to experience such tragedies in their late 40s to early 60s.

3. Cancer—loss of body parts such as one or both breasts, prostate issues or total removal, facial disfigurements, loss of inches of the intestines, colon, bladder, or part of the stomach essential for proper digestion. All are the possible results of various forms of cancer.

4. The inability of the body's appendages to elevate and/or maintain any elevation on command. This refers to your fingers, toes, or the most important appendage of the male body as described or understood by most males.

5. Having your chest cracked open while the surgeon performs bypass surgery, though s/he doesn't love you and might even come to the operating room drunk or drugged.

6. Extreme depression with thoughts or acts of suicide due to victimization by all the above losses. Why do I refer to patients as victims of those diseases? I do so because one becomes a victim if it involves loss of body parts or functions. For example, it is my sincere belief that the term "cancer survivor" focuses on and glamorizes the treatments for cancer while placing less emphasis on cures or prevention.

In a matter of speaking, I am a cancer survivor because I survive cancer on a daily basis. My DNA is attacked by 10,000 different free radicals or cancer-causing agents daily, but I intend to remain a survivor by not giving in to "eating in moderation" and compromising my physiological line of defense. I maintain my current healthy or "extreme" lifestyle only because I am a realist and I have witnessed time and time again the product of ignorant or irresponsible dietary behavior. What is even more shocking is to watch the so-called "health care professionals" fall victim to the same diseases they treat every day. And treat is all they do!

So, who needs this book? Those who currently follow the Standard American Diet (SAD), who believe wellness comes from fitness, and who live in America. All of those people groups desperately need this book. In fact, all of humanity needs this book no matter where you live or what you're eating these days.

This book is also for the physicians who prescribe harmful medications and the surgeons who have made an excellent living amputating limbs, excising, and re-routing organs and other body parts. And before or after retirement, they, too, will become dependent on the same medications they prescribed to manage diseases; and they will end up losing the same body parts and functions they surgically destroyed because of the poor dietary lifestyle that enriched them.

This book will benefit the judges who preside over trials and are easily irritated because they are suffering from diabetic conditions, sleep disorders, chronic pain, sexual dysfunctions, digestive disorders and/or constipation. All of those conditions are the foundation of their impotence and failure to think clearly, to rule on a matter effectively, and give up on life much too early. And it will also benefit religious leaders who have succumbed to the demon of gluttony.

Finally, this book is for the obese and out-of-shape professionals who are unable to carry out their duties effectively—the physicians, physical therapists, registered dieticians, nurses, hospital CEOs, school teachers, counselors, parents, police officers, firefighters, and anyone who plays an important part in a child's life. Their number one responsibility is to be a positive role model in the community, but too often they fail to do so. The truth is that your degrees and expertise in your respective fields will be rendered insignificant and eventually useless if you choose to follow a poor dietary lifestyle.

Here's a case in point. As a wellness instructor at a local hospital, I would often be asked by nurses or other employees my opinion about the nutritional qualities of certain food groups, often while in the presence of an obese registered dietitian. I thought these were set-ups to get me to undermine their credibility and professional authority, but "if the shoe fits, wear it." I couldn't be politically correct, but I was honest because to do otherwise would have been counter-productive and violate my own sense of integrity.

Our community leaders must operate the same way—with integrity—because they were elected, appointed, or selected to lead, not follow the pack. Respect must be earned, and once that happens, it must be maintained until you have a right to expect it.

Back To Health America is based on years of observation and interaction with patients and ordinary people who do and believe all of the above, which led me to the conclusion that "You are what you eat." No one needs to be a physician or dietician to understand that.

My passion and responsibility is to communicate wellness to all demographics. I feel compelled to break ranks and start a diet revolution that brings the government-medical-pharmaceutical-insurance complex to its knees, along with the health and fitness industries. The financial survival of all aforementioned groups depends on keeping people chemically dependent on medications, fitness programs, and dangerous foods—cooked dishes comprised of animal protein and processed carbohydrates—via slick, massive advertising campaigns and ease of availability.

I am unalterably opposed to and have never recommended eating a diet dominated by cooked and/or processed foods during my career. I walk the walk and talk the talk when I recommend a modified raw food diet to those who attend my seminars or other seminars at businesses, healthcare facilities, hospitals and schools in which I have taught.

Documented results from hospital staff, medical professionals, and patients suffering from diet-related diseases attest to reversing a smorgasbord of conditions by following my lifestyle recommendations. I also had several opportunities over the years to present my program at different professional venues. Letters came from a hospital, a law office, a chemical company, and an energy company.

As you read through this book, you will find several Life Lessons that contain portions of the many letters and cards I have received thanking me for telling them the truth. I have not incorporated them into this book to tout my wellness program. Instead, you will read about people of courage who became responsible and were willing to give my ideas a try and who might inspire you to take a chance. They were included in this book because it's the best way I know to honor them. They are my heroes—the folks who decided it was time to stop being exploited—the ones who had the vision to look beyond the traditional, climb out of their unhealthy boxes, and start living well for the first time in their lives. They wanted to stop being exploited and start living their lives with abundant health.

I have a message to share and a duty to my Creator. So do you. As individuals, we are ultimately responsible for our health and welfare. Take the questionnaire first, and then read the book. The only thing you will lose by not doing so is your health and wellness.

Questionnaire

If you answer "yes" to any of the following questions, you need to read this book!

1. Do you suffer from or take medication to treat indigestion?
2. Have you been diagnosed with Irritable Bowel Syndrome?
3. Do you suffer from recurrent stomach ulcers?
4. Have you been diagnosed with diverticulitis?
5. Has your gallbladder been removed?
6. Do you follow a low-fat diet and still gain weight?
7. Are you or your children fat?
8. Are your clothes getting smaller?
9. Do you drink 7-8 glasses of water daily to hydrate your body/ promote weight loss?
10. Do you trust the surgeon to tell you the whole truth before a gastric bypass?
11. Do you suffer from or take medication to treat frequent constipation or diarrhea?
12. Do you have, or have you had, kidney stones?
13. Do you run out of energy easily?
14. Do you nap frequently or fall asleep at work, meetings or behind the wheel?

15. Has your spouse asked you to sleep in another room because you snore?
16. Do you suffer from sleep apnea?
17. Do you drink, take medication or wear a breathing device to go to sleep?
18. Do you suffer from iron deficiency?
19. Do you suffer with episodic dizziness or weakness?
20. Are you frequently irritable?
21. Do you often drink tea, soda, coffee, or power drinks to boost energy?
22. Do you eat at fast-food franchises more than once a week?
23. Do you believe regular exercise is the answer to good health?
24. Do you believe wellness is achieved through fitness?
25. Do you suffer from or take medication to treat low back pain?
26. Have you had muscle or joint pain, lasting over six weeks that required a physician's attention?
27. Do you smoke, drink, eat or take medication to deal with stress?
28. Do you suffer from or take medication to deal with depression?
29. Do you suffer from or take medication to treat sinusitis?
30. Do you suffer from/take medication to treat recurrent 24-hour viruses or bugs?
31. Do you take medication to treat high blood pressure, triglycerides or diabetes?
32. Do you suffer from or take medication to treat sexual dysfunction?
33. Do you believe drug companies have your best interests in mind?
34. Do you drink soda more than once a week?
35. Do you believe vitamin supplements are the answer to good health?
36. Do you believe dairy products provide calcium and Vitamin D/ prevent osteoporosis?
37. Do you believe meat, fish, chicken, nuts or cooked beans are healthy sources of protein?
38. Do you believe everyone's needs are different to improve his/ her health?

39. Do you depend on New Year's resolutions to improve your health?
40. Do you believe eating everything in moderation/using portion control is healthy?
41. Do you believe nutritional labels as the gospel truth?
42. Have you been diagnosed with any form of cancer?
43. Have you ever had a skin lesion or cancer removed from your body?
44. Do you believe the FDA and USDA have your best interests in mind?
45. Should you always believe or trust the health advice of the "healthcare professionals?"
46. Do you suffer from excess bleeding during your menstrual cycle?
47. Do you suffer from excessive cramping during your menstrual cycle?

The Great **Equalizer**

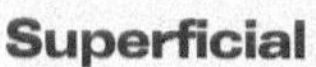

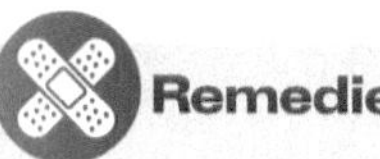

0-30 years of age

Occasional colds, flu, pneumonia, viruses, diarrhea, constipation, allergies, headaches, snoring, weight gain, irritability, decreased energy, insomnia, urinary tract infections, hypoglycemia, severe menstrual cramps, kidney stones & generalized aches.

→ Occasional Doctor visits, prescriptions & over-the-counter drugs, supplements. Attempting various diets and exercise/fitness programs.

30-45 years of age

Kidney stones, joint pain, low back pain, fainting, migraines, gallbladder & other digestive diseases, obesity, hypertension, high blood fat, hyperglycemia, atrial fibrillation, sleep apnea, gout, sexual dysfunction.

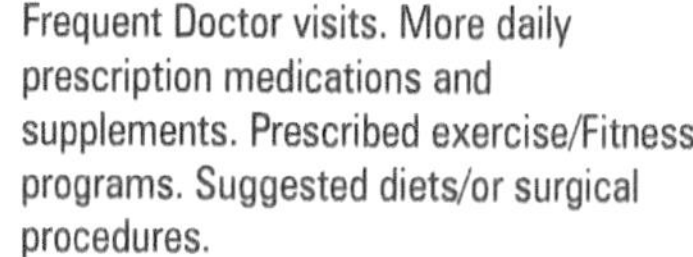

→ Frequent Doctor visits. More daily prescription medications and supplements. Prescribed exercise/Fitness programs. Suggested diets/or surgical procedures.

45-55 years of age

Drug dependency/side effects, degenerative join/disc disease, sluggishness, insomnia, poor energy, frequent work absenteeism due to hyperglycemia/hypertension & side effects. Dietary & physical limitations.

→ Increased Doctor visits. Joint replacements, various surgeries, hospitalizations, forced early retirement. Prescribed and mandatory exercise/fitness & diet regimen. Increased number of potent prescription drugs & supplements.

55-80 years of age

CANCER	STROKE	HEART ATTACK	DIABETES	ALZHEIMER'S
Loss of hair, appetite, body parts/organs, Chemo & Radiation	Paralysis, difficulty walking, speech and vision impairment	Shortness of breath, functional limitation, poor endurance	Loss of sight & limbs, vascular/heart diseases, neuropathy	Memory loss, no recognition of family members, total dependency

Functional and dietary limitations. Severe drug dependencies/side effects, depression, coping with serious diseases & handicaps. Family or outside agency dependency. Skilled nursing facility placement.

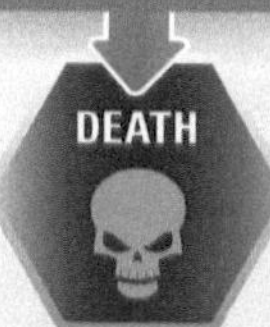

Chapter 1

A Personal Journey to Wellness

The Foundation

How we get to where we are is harder for some than for others, and vice versa. Our lives may be filled with the best intentions, the greatest ideals, and a sprinkling of dreams, but life is full of twists and turns that often lead us down roads we didn't look for or that must be explored. It has been no different for me—a journey to wellness I never anticipated. My story is long and likely different from anything experienced by most Americans, but it must be told.

I grew up in a three-room house in Abadan, a small town in the central western region of Iran that is separated from the Iraqi border by the Karun River. At one time, Abadan was a marketplace for salt and woven mats but it's now home to the second largest oil refinery in the world. This made it the target of some of the most intense bombing of the 1980 Iran-Iraq War, which started one year after I came to America as a teenager.

I did not grow up in the desert and only saw a camel at the zoo. I was considered a city boy—the son of a machinist who worked for the oil company at the local technical college. My mother was a very kind homemaker who often borrowed money to help strangers in need when we had very little of it ourselves. Still, she took good care of me, my two younger sisters and my older brother.

Education was important to my parents. When I was in middle school, I attended classes six days a week. I studied biology, chemistry, algebra, geometry, new math, physical education, geography and history, as well as English, Persian, Arabic, and Industrial Arts. School was serious business. I loved studying English and being around Americans, who seemed to share and enjoy my sense of humor. I would often go to work with my dad who constructed, with precision, various metal and wooden devices used educationally by American instructors at the college.

Because I loved English so much, my father would sometimes bring me American or English books borrowed from co-workers. I would study them for hours and would actually speak English in my sleep, or so my mother told me. Clearly my education was an integral part of my journey to wellness; but so was life experience.

When I was around 10 years old, things began to unravel. My father did not work out at a gym, but he had muscular arms and broad shoulders. Unfortunately, he was an alcoholic who would often come home drunk. My friends made fun of him and, to save face, I would sometimes join them. It was not so easy for my brother, Javid. One day he saw a police officer brutally beating a drunken citizen. Totally traumatized by what he saw revealed that he was suffering from several psychological issues and was near an emotional breakdown. My father promised God that he would stop drinking if my brother's health improved.

Javid went to various psychiatrists who put him on medications that only made his mental state worse. Some put him in a psychological fog, something I would later see many times in my healthcare career in America. Finally, my father decided that enough was enough and threw away the prescriptions. Gradually, my brother got well and my father kept his promise to God—he went cold turkey and gave up drinking.

That's when my father started paying more attention to health and wellness for himself and his family. Prior to my father's transformation, we ate mostly chicken, fish, lamb, and rice, and often finished our meals with sweets. A typical breakfast consisted of scrambled eggs, butter, bread, and feta or cream cheese along with hot tea. Sometimes my father would raise a lamb in the back yard and then kill it for my mother to clean. The next morning, we would have boiled sheep's head, hooves, and stomach. Back then, I considered it a most delicious meal. Now, I cannot imagine how I ate it. Oddly, I never cared much for the taste of beef, not even in Iran, which was just a matter of personal taste.

My father believed as most do that only meat could provide certain critical nutrients. Nevertheless, he started eating more vegetables and other plant-based foods. For breakfast, he consumed raw garlic with cilantro or green onions with bread. I now know that when slicing or crushing garlic, its natural enzymes turn into allicin, an organosulfur compound responsible for its strong odor. Years later, I learned that allicin is used for its antimicrobial properties. I also learned that garlic loses its nutritional value about two or three hours after you cut it which means taking garlic powder or capsules is useless.

Thanks to my father's new health habits, he lost the belly fat he accrued during his early 30s. My mother, who was in charge of the cooking, didn't eat as healthy, and my father often scolded her for using too much salt, fat and grease in our food. Unlike my dad, she was sick a lot. Now 73, she has diabetes, high blood pressure, neuropathy and swelling of the ankles, and she often loses her balance and falls. Until recently, my 81-year-old father continued to ride his bike out of town for six hours at a time. My brother, only two years older than me, has had several back surgeries and doctors have told him that his carotid arteries are clogged. My sisters, who are in their 40s, are both overweight and have problems with their feet. My father fared far better than my mother or my siblings. They would have been wise and a great deal healthier had they adopted my father's ideas on healthy eating.

Leaving for America

In 1978, the Iranian people began protesting the reign of Mohammad Reza Shah Pahlavi, known simply as the Shah, a heavy-handed dictator who appeared to be out of touch with lower-class families like mine. Those who said anything against his regime usually disappeared. Eventually, he was replaced by the Ayatollah Khomeini, the leader of the Revolution, and many lost their lives fighting for or against the political changes.

Things went from bad to worse. The schools were closed for almost two years during the revolt. At fifteen, I watched at night as my friends threw rocks at the police, who retaliated with bullets. When one of my friends was shot in the head and died, I begged my father to send me to America to finish my education. I was the only one of my siblings doing fairly well in school while trying to stay out of trouble. My father saw my potential to succeed which led him to withdraw half his savings from the bank—savings he had amassed while working days as a machinist and nights as a taxi driver, transporting passengers out of town in his own car. I have been one of my father's best investment.

In January of 1979, I traveled alone for the first time from Abadan with five thousand dollars in cash and travelers checks stuffed in my pocket. I was terrified, especially when I lost my passport in the London airport. Although I spoke the King's English I learned at school, I couldn't communicate with airport security. I cried like a baby until someone found an Iranian employee to translate for me. We retraced my steps until we found the missing passport. That man became my friend for life and I was able to continue my journey to America.

The Next Leg of the Journey

I was picked up at Hartsfield International Airport in Atlanta by my uncle, six years my senior, and we headed to Chattanooga where we shared an apartment. I enrolled in high school a week later, but it wasn't easy coping with the change in cultures. Though I excelled in English classes in Iran, it was difficult for me to handle English spoken with a Southern accent. Some days I would come home crying because I couldn't understand some of the words my classmates and teachers said. Other times, I was just puzzled by Southern lingo like, "You come back, you hear?" As far as I knew, my hearing was just fine. Of course my name, Jamshid, was another source of humor for my classmates. "That sounds like what you say when you step on something," one of my friends once told me. When I became an American citizen, I legally added James as my middle name. It was easier that way. I was culturally correct.

Six months after arriving in Chattanooga, I was out of money. Some was used for our living expenses and some was used for my uncle's college tuition. I took a job as a janitor and lawn man at First Baptist Church, which was my uncle's idea. He'd been offered the job, but talked me into taking it to help pay the bills. He promised that he would help me finish school after he graduated. It never happened. I supported the two of us for over a year while attending high school but when my uncle completed his studies, he went to Texas and I was left alone to fend for myself. Relatives don't always come through as they promise.

The College Years

The loss of two years of school in Iran didn't stop me from earning my high school diploma when I was seventeen. I was ahead of my classmates in Tennessee and continued my studies at Chattanooga State. My friends urged me to study computer science, which bored me to death. Since college took up most of my day, I could no longer work full time or afford a place of my own. I stayed with various acquaintances who were gracious enough to welcome me into their homes for a few months at a time. One of them, a wealthy retired teacher with a disability, hired me to drive her around and help with odd chores. Her husband had suffered a stroke and was living at a nearby nursing home, and I often took her to visit him. That's where and when I saw physical therapists at work for the first time.

There was something about the healing movements and the interaction with the stroke patients that sparked my curiosity. I love people, but I've always clicked with older people partly because I missed my parents and grandmother so much when I left Iran. Suddenly I had a plan for my education and my future—but not so fast. I talked with my academic adviser and began taking the necessary prerequisites to become a physical therapist. However, the only physical therapy school in Tennessee was in Memphis, six hours away. My grades were okay, but the program was highly competitive and my application was denied. I went on and earned a Bachelor of Science in Biology at the University of Tennessee at Chattanooga, then re-enrolled at Chattanooga State and became a licensed physical therapist assistant.

The New Career and New Ideas

My education allowed me to work hands-on with patients, but I was not allowed to evaluate them and create their care plans. I also worked two jobs to provide for my then-wife and five-year-old daughter, Shereen. Mornings were spent helping patients in nursing homes in Dalton, Georgia; afternoons and evenings were spent working with another group at Memorial Hospital in Chattanooga. I did this for several years before working in home health care and at other nursing homes. Eventually I conducted wellness classes and therapy sessions at Erlanger Medical Center, an academic and trauma care hospital in Chattanooga.

It didn't take long for me to make the connection between diet and disease. At the nursing homes, I noticed that almost every patient with Alzheimer's or other forms of dementia also suffered from either diabetes or high blood pressure. It is well known that diabetes and high blood pressure are caused by poor dietary habits, so maybe the same was true for dementia. When I voiced this idea to my co-workers, they laughed at me and opined that Alzheimer's is either genetic or is caused by drinking out of aluminum cans. I didn't buy it.

It is widely known that poor nutrition can and often does lead to diabetes, which causes neuropathy (poor sensation or nerve problems/damage in the extremities). Therefore, one can also conclude that poor nutrition, over time, can cripple a person's thought processes due to misfiring of the neurons in the brain. Remember, the brain is an organ that needs nutrient-dense blood to work properly. If you give it junk, it will get gummed up with that junk until it is cleansed out of the body. My ideas were validated while working at Memorial Hospital where I met a physical therapist co-worker who was Seventh-day Adventist. I was intrigued by some of the foods she brought for lunch, especially the meat substitutes, and started questioning her about her eating habits. I experimented by stopping all beef consumption and my energy level immediately went up. There was something to my ideas about diet and physical wellness and I was determined to get to the bottom of what is actually a well-kept secret.

My Diet Evolution

When I was a teenager I suffered from seasonal pollen allergies, even in Iran. If I didn't take the antihistamines prescribed by doctors, I would have to live with sneezing, watery eyes and a runny nose. When spring and fall allergy seasons started, I would suffer for a week, but I never lost workdays. I wondered if my diet contributed to the onset of my allergies.

About ten years after I started practicing as a physical therapist assistant, I gave up chicken and dairy products to see if I could improve my health even more. At the time, I weighed 165 pounds, which was too much weight for my five-foot-five-inch frame. I jogged five miles every other day, but my weight stayed the same until I changed my eating habits. The first month after I stopped eating chicken, cheese, milk and other dairy products, I lost ten pounds and my allergies went away. Spring allergy season was fast approaching, but I barely noticed its arrival.

Then I remembered when I first became allergic to tree and grass pollen. At my middle school in Iran, school officials started serving small cartons of fortified milk with our lunches, which we ate in the classroom. I never drank milk on a regular basis because we always had tea at home. Cheese, too, began to appear on our lunch plates—slices of cheddar carved from huge blocks. The dairy products were intended to supplement the nutrition we were receiving at home, but the side effects were awful. Once I saw the connection, I gradually eliminated most processed items from my diet and felt even better. Now it was time to see what would happen if my patients, many of whom had multiple medical problems, gave up the same unhealthy foods.

Albert's Story

At fifty-four, morbidly-obese Albert was recovering from a stroke at a local nursing home in Chattanooga, Tennessee. He was so huge that I was the only one in the whole department who could get him in and out of bed. Not only was I strong, I used the proper technique and gave Albert time to trust me. Like many of the other patients, Albert had diabetes and high blood pressure. The stroke had left him flaccid on one side of his body, and he couldn't walk.

I had earned a reputation for never showing signs of fatigue, even after long hours on the job. One day he asked me where I got all my energy. I explained that I eat only fresh fruits and vegetables whenever possible—no meat, no dairy, no processed foods from a box. This was in direct opposition to Albert's diet. When his family came to visit, they brought him cookies and other high-calorie sweets. I encouraged them to bring him fruit instead.

Albert lamented that his nutritionist cautioned him about fruit because of the sugar content and that the diet she prescribed was the only way to get his weight down. When I asked Albert if he believed her, he experienced a dose of reality and stated that she was extremely overweight and had her own health problems. Albert realized she couldn't help him, but I could.

I was not a nutritionist, but I was trim and in excellent health, something Albert could see for himself. That made me a good representative for what I said and did.

When I realized that Albert didn't like the nursing home food and refused to eat it, I asked him if he would eat food I prepared for him at home. He said he would pretend to eat what they served him but eat my dishes instead when the nurses weren't looking; and his family agreed to the plan. My shifts at the nursing home were seven or eight hours long. I would get Albert up in the morning, help him get dressed and put him to bed in the evening. I brought him plant-based meals and snacks from home and monitored his food intake and activities. Six months later, Albert had lost forty pounds, his diabetes and high blood pressure were under control, and he was walking with a quad cane.

Albert began to feel independent again and made plans to live with his 400-pound sister who smoked—a disaster in the making. I warned him that he would start smoking again and resume his old eating habits. He promised me he would take care of himself, but he didn't. Four months after he left the nursing home, Albert was in the emergency room with congestive heart failure, and I went to see him. He passed away at age fifty-five. I wish I had more time with Albert because I saw how my dietary suggestions had improved his quality of life.

My experience with Albert strengthened my resolve to promote responsible eating whenever I could; and I continued to do the same for myself. I deleted other items from my diet such as nuts and other processed foods to see what would happen. I was consuming seventy-five percent raw foods, twenty-five percent cooked foods, and eating out three or four times a week. I changed this to a raw food intake of ninety-five percent and one weekly restaurant meal while educating myself on the natural medicinal properties of fruits and vegetables. For example, apples are packed with nutrients that can absorb oils and other stomach-upsetting ingredients and get rid of indigestion. I was getting healthier by the minute.

Life Stresses, Traumas and Other Intrusions

I am convinced that my plantarian lifestyle protected me from health problems during two very stressful times in my life—health problems that often affect people who are dealing with stress or trauma. In 2000, my wife and I divorced and she kept the house. The financial demands of the legal proceedings, child support, and tuition for my son's private school depleted my funds and left me homeless for more than a year. Sometimes I slept in my car; other nights, I slept at the hospital where I was working.

During a divorce, many people become depressed, which causes too much weight loss from not eating enough or excessive weight gain from consuming "comfort foods." Since they don't eat the right types of foods, their overall health begins to decline and they experience a variety of problems in addition to the ones they're already facing. I was determined not to let this happen to me. I focused even more on my nutrition, and made sure I ate plenty of raw fruits and vegetables that would bolster my immune system and ward off stress-related illnesses. To the surprise of my co-workers, I became the most productive and healthiest member of the physical therapy department.

Ten years later, I went from the proverbial frying pan into the fire. I tried to help a friend purchase a house, but when she failed to make the house payments I wound up entangled in a three-year legal battle that cost me a great deal of money. My friend's betrayal and the resulting financial loss almost destroyed me, but I knew I had to take care of myself. Again, I consumed even more raw fruits and vegetables than usual and, again, I stayed healthy. Good nutrition is always the first line of defense against illness, even in tough times.

I wasn't wise about my finances, protecting my savings, or making a wise investment, but I did learn how to invest in the well-being of my physical body. With each step, each investment, my health got better and better. When I talk to people my age, some of whom are quite wealthy and successful, they all seem to be suffering from some disease or symptom I wasn't experiencing—fatigue, hemorrhoids, constipation, kidney stones, headaches, joint pain, diabetes, sleep apnea, high blood pressure, snoring, irritability and sexual dysfunction—so I knew I was on the right track. When I walk in a room, those same people want to know what Albert wanted to know. They are amazed by my level of energy and why I am happy even in the face of disaster. The truth is, they wanted it, too!

Coming Full Circle

I now practice physical therapy at a senior retirement complex and my good health continues to intrigue the patients I see. I often bring them a breakfast of seasonal fruit and encourage them to adopt a healthier, plantarian lifestyle. When they do, they see their blood sugar return to normal and their blood pressure drops every time. Sometimes peer pressure or family influence takes over and they go back to their old eating habits; but as long as they stick to a pure, plant-based diet, they get results. It doesn't take long for them to feel better and more energetic, no matter how old they are or how long they've been in poor health.

After seeing how much my patients benefited from my plantarian lifestyle despite their ages, medical conditions, and lifelong eating habits, I thought about getting a degree in nutrition. However, I couldn't devote two years of my life learning concepts that do not work or becoming part of a group of healthcare professionals who are not healthy. At the hospitals where I was employed, the staff nutritionists were obese and/or diabetic, had high blood pressure or cancer—serious conditions that are all related to poor nutritional lifestyle. The one who had juvenile diabetes talked to patients as if she was proud of it and told them how she controlled her blood sugar, but she never told them about ways to reverse the disease. Ironically, her advice didn't work.

Likewise, a lot of researchers are studying why some people get cancer, or what route diabetes takes and how to control it once it's diagnosed. It's like studying a drunk driver's behavior to see if he ends up hitting a pole or veering off into a ditch. If he doesn't drink and get behind the wheel, neither is going to happen. The same is true for, i.e., cancer or diabetes. It doesn't matter if your life ends with a particular disease or the route the disease took to kill you. If you know how to prevent the disease, you won't need a flawed road map because the end will be much farther down a healthier road. Even the experts don't know that much about nutrition. They're required to follow and protect certain guidelines and tell you about them. If they don't follow the popular diet game plan of the day, they risk alienation within their professions.

This book is not about nutrition; it is about behavior. You don't need in-depth nutritional counseling or scientific studies. Once you know which foods improve your health, you simply eat those foods to stay healthy. Otherwise, you're acting irresponsibly with your own body just like the drunk driver who will eventually hit a telephone pole, crash into a ditch, or worse. Because this book contradicts mainstream healthcare, nutrition, and medicine, I hope you will read it with an open mind. The proof is not just in how well my patients feel when they adopt this lifestyle, but in the indisputable changes that follow: lower blood pressure, cholesterol and blood sugar; the reversal of heart problems and other life-threatening conditions; and a decreased need for expensive and harmful medications. I am living proof that it works, and so are they.

Chapter 2

Wellness Accountability

What is food?

When I looked up the definition of food, I was not surprised to find that almost all Internet sites defined it as just about any "nutritious substance" absorbed by plants or that is eaten or ingested by people or animals so they stay alive and grow. Of course, almost all of those sites made it clear that food comes from plants or animals.

My definition of food is very complete. Food is any nutritious substance, consisting of macronutrients such as fats, protein and carbohydrates, and micronutrients such as enzymes, minerals and vitamins that people, animals or plants ingest or absorb in order to maintain life, repair tissue damage, and produce energy and growth. In order for the food to be digested without any harmful side effects, it must consist of all of the above nutrients in the right balance; and only nature—as in vines, bushes and trees—is capable of producing that balance.

Digestible or Indigestible?

Some substances are digestible and others are indigestible. Digestible substances are those that contain all the nutrients in the right balance that support and facilitate the digestion process, and promote life sustaining fuel and vitality to all the cells, tissues, organs, and systems of the body. Indigestible substances are "foods" that have all the nutrients depleted from them through exposure to extreme heat, e.g., cooking processes, juicing, drying, or chemical alteration. Those substances tend to lose their nutritional strength and balance and can no longer effectively defend the body against foreign invaders, such as flu, other viruses, bacterial invasions, cancers, and other diseases or syndromes. An indigestible substance typically relies on the body's reserve nutrients such as vitamins, minerals, and enzymes to be digested.

There are consequences that accrue from ingesting indigestible substances. I have worked in all the hospitals and many homes in town as well as those in surrounding cities. My job and focus has always been to provide healthcare services to my patients, and since I'm involved primarily in physical therapy, I have witnessed the consequences of repeated drunk driving. I have also seen what happens to our bodies when we regularly consume indigestible substances every day. It's not a pretty picture. Throughout my studies and experiments with different clients, I have learned that only major behavioral changes that incorporate choosing to eat digestible substances will lead to a reversal of the destructive reactions produced by the human body.

Life Lesson—Dan's Double Chins

Dan, a doctor of physical therapy, worked with me on a healthy lifestyle for about 18 months. He always believed he was health conscious, stayed active and strong, and rarely got sick. However, he knew there was something missing. He wrote, "Though no one ever mentioned my weight or my looks, actually stating that I looked good, I had ballooned up to 225 pounds two years ago. With a six-foot-one-inch frame and an athletic build at age 29, that was borderline obese according to health standards." Dan's diet at work started to take its toll on him, producing swollen cheeks and double chins. "I decided to make a change and was lucky enough to receive your help and council at that time. I listened to your explanations, questioned your theories (which I still do), implemented your program, and here I am, as healthy as ever and 45 pounds lighter. I can only imagine the ways in which my body must be thanking me." Dan had less degeneration, improved circulation, and reduced damage to his vital organs and the vessels of his body. He changed his lifestyle and brought those changes to his family, which made it an outstanding journey to wellness.

Mythical Immunity

No one is immune from an unhealthy diet, no matter what their occupation or status in life. Accountants, men of God, judges, attorneys, surgeons, mechanics, physicians, musicians, nurses, teachers, children, successful investors, scientists, town drunks, and even homeless individuals may all have unhealthy diets in common. Their financial soundness or lack thereof, educational achievements or lack of them, their spiritual wealth or poverty, their political affiliations or connections make no difference in their ability to fight diseases and their outcomes. They all seem to end up in hospital beds dealing with the same chronic ailments.

We have been given free will to choose our path in life and we live and die by our choices. I have witnessed people of different walks of life, socioeconomic and educational backgrounds victimized by the poor choices of ingestible substances. Those people are not survivors, by any means.

Here's the real truth about what to eat and what not to eat. The foods you eat provide your body with "information" and substances needed to function properly (Denton, 2013). If your body doesn't get the correct information, your metabolic processes will suffer and your health will begin to fail. Consuming too much of the wrong foods provides your body with inaccurate instructions, which leads to weight gain, lack of nourishment, and a high risk for incurring diseases and/or conditions like arthritis, diabetes, different forms of cancer, and heart disease. What we eat and how much of it we eat determines the level of our health and the intensity of our journey to wellness.

Playing the Blame Game

You can convince yourself that your health problems are inherited, caused by your spouse or children, your occupation, or that it's just God's plan for your life, especially when things don't work as you wish they would. While some of those are somewhat rightfully "easy to blame," the buck stops with you. You know if you're eating unhealthy or indigestible foods just as you know how harmful those substances are for your body. That means taking responsibility for your eating habits and not blaming the folks who manufacture those indigestible products they label as food. If you are totally ignorant regarding proper and responsible dietary habits, this book will hopefully make you wiser and more aware of the truth about how to achieve and maintain true wellness. So let's go one step further.

The truth is that it's very difficult to discuss health and wellness accountability without first addressing "political correctness," which has paralyzed our nation and trampled our right to freedom of speech. When I think of wellness accountability and political correctness, I must admit my mind conjures up images of one of the most influential and well-known women in the world—a woman who has encouraged and motivated many individuals. She has inspired women from all walks of life to stand up for their rights and fight for their freedom in all endeavors; and she's done so much more. She has promoted and given rise to people who claim to have health, wellness, and your best medical interests at heart, but who have contributed very little to the true definition of wellness. Unfortunately, their rise to fame has included urging many unsuspecting people to walk down the wrong paths toward their ideas of wellness.

Celebrities Are No Exception

In December 2014, during a televised interview led by a powerhouse of journalism, this influential celebrity was asked to choose the most important goal she hadn't achieved yet, even though she has everything anyone could want at age 60. She stated that she would like to be at peace with her weight. I suppose that those who've wrestled with excessive poundage for most of their lives would like to have the same type of peace to which she referred, but it's not a great idea and it's a false peace.

Having peace, being content, or giving in to issues of excess body weight is the same as being at peace with all the maladies associated with poor health and lifestyle choices that also lead to weight gain and obesity. Here's a woman who has everything financially as well as the respect of millions around the world, but she still struggles to understand or attain one simple goal—good health and true wellness.

Unfortunately, her influential, role-model status and her response to the interviewer's question sent the wrong and misleading message to millions of people, especially women who often struggle with their own weight and health issues. While the question that was posed to her was tough to answer, she did not arm those hoping for genuine pearls of wisdom with sound health advice—the most important wisdom for anyone to live a life of true wellness.

Add to that the many fitness trainers who have helped her lose weight, which she has sometimes achieved, and the problem remains the same—loss of weight without ever achieving wellness. Her journey there has become so circular, filled with wrong information and advice, and dependent on fitness trainers and gym attendance that didn't work, that she has now accepted her current condition. Even one of her best cardiologist pals has not been able to make a difference in her health because he was either politically correct or just afraid to tell her the truth. That's not the way I operate. She may be influential and powerful, but I am compelled to tell her the truth. The truth in wellness as I know it will give her freedom from ignorance, myths, and lies so she may be able to continue with her good deeds and inspirations—and all of you as well—with no regard for political correctness. "If you don't eat the way others eat, your health and weight will normalize and be your own, not that of someone else."

With that in mind, it's easy to blame food producers/manufacturers just as we blame all the others on the list above, but it's still wrong. No one is forcing you to buy products you know lack nutrients and are bad for your body. Look at the products in your pantry or food cabinets. Check out what's lurking in your refrigerator and freezer. By taking inventory of what you purchase, you will understand how you support the very companies you blame for all your ills. If you buy several 12-packs of soda in cans or bottles and drink those caffeine and sugar-laden drinks, you did so voluntarily. Foods and drinks that are filled with high levels of simple sugars, preservatives, and other nasty ingredients wouldn't be on the grocery shelves if people refused to buy them (Clower, 2014).

The same holds true for foods containing trans-fats. It's ironic that the guidelines for low-fat intake were published at approximately the same time the obesity epidemic began—around 1977 (Gunnars, 2012-2014). Consider also that most of the Omega-6 fats you consume are a fatty acid known as linoleic acid. Is it good for you? Studies show that this fatty acid, which gets incorporated into your cell membranes and body fat stores, is likely to oxidize, leading to damaged molecules such as DNA and an increase in the risk of cancer. So much for all those healthy processed vegetable oils; it's best to let them stay on the grocery shelves instead of occupying space in your pantry or finding their way into your diet. If we don't buy them, the companies that pawn them off on us with all kinds of health lies will stop making them.

Intoxicating and Indigestible

I am extremely concerned that we are deliberately or ignorantly impairing our health, and that's what an alcoholic does—impairs his/her body. Think about what happens when you drink alcoholic beverages. The body metabolizes alcohol very fast and, unlike food, needs no time for digestion. It is also absorbed before almost all other nutrients - it takes about about 60 seconds for alcohol to reach the brain because approximately 20 percent is absorbed across the walls of an empty stomach (Alcohol and Your Health, 2014). Every organ of the body is affected by alcohol consumption, but the liver takes most of the brunt. Liver cells need healthy fatty acids for fuel, then send triglycerides to other body tissues. But alcohol gets to the head of the metabolic line, which results in the accumulation of fatty acids and lasting changes to the structure of liver cells, impairing the cells' ability to metabolize fats (Alcohol and Your Health, 2014). This is why consumption of alcohol, especially via heavy drinking, can lead to injury to the body and the death of impaired drivers and/or others (Alcohol and Your Health, 2014).

Alcohol is a toxin and consumption also leads to malnutrition. Since alcohol is processed by the digestive system, it competes with a limited amount of nutritional resources that usually provide the body with nourishment. The brain and nervous system are the first to be affected and, within minutes of consumption, the affects become apparent with regard to judgment, sensory perceptions, and muscle coordination (Smith, 2012). As noted above, the liver processes alcohol, which affects steady blood sugar levels. Those at risk for diabetes or who already have the disease could find themselves in a diabetic crisis from drinking alcohol (Smith, 2012).

Alcohol suppresses hunger and also aggravates the lining of the stomach and small intestines by increasing acid secretion and blocking the body's ability to absorb essential nutrients from healthier foods, which leads to malnutrition and/or anemia (Smith, 2012). This includes the loss of niacin, B-1 (thiamine), and other B vitamins that must be used by the liver to metabolize alcohol. This leads to less absorption and storage of B-12 and folacin, as well as the dumping of high amounts of vitamin A into the blood stream, which causes sharp vision at first and then night blindness (Smith, 2012). Lastly, alcohol is a diuretic, which leads to greater output of urine. When that happens, the body loses water-soluble minerals including zinc, potassium, and magnesium (Smith, 2012).

It's in this condition that many drivers get behind the wheel of an automobile and attempt to drive normally. Most cultures have a very dim view of intoxicated drivers. We tend to have less understanding and compassion for them. In most cases, we believe they should be held legally responsible and incur monetary fines and/or jail time. In some cases, we find ourselves saying, "They deserve to get what's coming to them!" However, when a diabetic or a hypertensive driver experiences diabetic shock or a coma, a stroke, or a heart attack behind the wheel as a result of their own poor choices, we tend to be totally understanding and compassionate, even when such irresponsible behavior results in injuries or death to self and/or others.

More often than not, those who survive are sent to the hospital for treatment while we pray for their speedy recovery, even though we know the accident in which they were involved was the result of medical conditions created by the irresponsible ingestion of indigestible substances. The drunk driver and the driver suffering from specific illnesses create havoc in their own lives and the lives of others as a result of their irresponsible actions, but they are judged differently by society and law makers. Is it a double standard or ignorance? Maybe it's a lot of both.

Mental/Emotional Impairments and Diet

Many people suffer endlessly from mental and emotional impairments that can be helped via a plantarian diet. Since food provides necessary nourishment for the mind and body, it is beyond wise to provide loved ones and yourself with the nutrition needed to keep the body energized and in optimal working condition. The brain receives incoming nutrients before the rest of your body because it orchestrates all other body organs, cells, and metabolic processes (F.E, Dr., 2014). Small deficiencies of certain nutrients are ample enough to alter and affect mood and brain chemistry, especially in individuals who are sensitive (F.E, Dr., 2014). It's not surprising that the first consequences of nutritional deficiencies show up as mental health symptoms (Cass, 2014).

Whether you're an adult, a teenager, or a child, a physician can prescribe a variety of antidepressants and even herbs, but if nutritional deficiencies are the root cause, which they almost always are, no medication or herb will make a difference. For example, B vitamins appear to protect against atrophy of the brain and cognitive impairment (F.E, Dr., 2014). Omega-3 fatty acids are extremely important for brain health as well as mood improvement. Increasing certain nutrients may have a huge positive impact on mental health (F.E, Dr., 2014).

Today's diets contain almost no nutrition because the nutrition has been cooked out or processed out of food. We consume far too much sugar, not enough fiber, and dine on additives and preservatives - a sure-fire way for non-absorption of essential nutrients and poor nutrition (Cass, 2014). You can eat and eat until your stomach wants to burst and you will still be poorly nourished, which means your brain will receive little or no nourishment. There are several amino acids, vitamins, minerals, and other nutrients that are needed for good mental health. This includes fatty acids, which help prevent or treat depression and other mental/emotional disorders (Cass, 2014).

Here's how it works. If the brain's neurotransmitters (the messengers) are in need of reinforcements—think of needed troops in the military—depression can walk in and take over your mind and eventually your whole life. Amino acids are the foundation of protein and are needed by the neuro-transmitters. The three amino acids that affect mood and depression are phenylalanine, tyrosine, and tryptophan. Phenylalanine and tyrosine manufacture norepinephrine, a neurotransmitter, and tryptophan is eventually changed into serotonin. (Cass, 2014).

This is especially true for those who suffer from drug addictions. As noted above, serotonin is made from the amino acid tryptophan which is found in food. In order for this conversion to take place, the body must have many components from food including magnesium, vitamins B-6, B-12, vitamin D, folic acid, and zinc, to name just a few (Plesman, 2011). Most people find it hard to believe that drug addiction has anything to do with nutrition, but they're wrong. The nutritional requirements are extremely multifaceted and "supplementing with miracle nutrients such as vitamins and minerals" is not the answer (Plesman, 2011). Individuals on a diet that's low in protein and high in simple carbohydrates can't provide their bodies with the nutrients needed to produce the "feel good" transmitters, and each person has "a unique biochemical make-up" (Plesman, 2011).

We need the various nutritional forerunners of those "feel good" neurotransmitters and we must also have energy in order to change one group of molecules into another needed set. If the brain is starved for energy, it releases stress hormones such as adrenaline and cortisol, which change energy stores in the body (i.e. glycogen) to provide the brain with needed energy (Plesman, 2011). Unfortunately, those stress hormones may cause anxiety and nervousness, which leads a person to self-medicate using legal or illegal drugs (Plesman, 2011).

Vitamins from a plantarian diet are catalysts that help speed up chemical processes needed by the brain and for survival. Without vitamins, we can and often do slip into a depressive state because our brains don't have the healthy fuel needed to function. The brain uses Vitamin B1 (thiamine) to help convert glucose, or blood sugar, into fuel - without it the brain rapidly runs out of energy (Cass, 2014). "This can lead to fatigue, depression, irritability, anxiety, and even thoughts of suicide. Deficiencies can also cause memory problems, loss of appetite, insomnia, and gastrointestinal disorders" (Cass, 2014).

Here's a reality check: eating foods high in refined carbohydrates, such as simple sugars, use up the body's B1 supply. A niacin (vitamin B-3) deficiency causes Pellagra, an illness that produces psychosis and dementia (Cass, 2014). However, niacin deficiencies that are not clinical in nature are known to produce agitation and anxiety along with mental and physical slowness (Cass, 2014). The list of needed nutrients for mental health is no different than the list of what's needed by the body as a whole. Here are a few examples:

Pyridoxine (vitamin B-6) creates neurotransmitters that help prevent depression and a deficiency can lead to "anemia, numbness, tingling in the limbs, and convulsions" (Cass, 2014). Vitamin B-12 (cobalamin) helps create red blood cells and transport oxygen. Without it, you can suffer from pernicious anemia, which can cause "mood swings, paranoia, irritability, confusion, dementia, hallucinations, or mania, eventually followed by appetite loss, dizziness, weakness, shortage of breath, heart palpitations, diarrhea, and tingling sensations in the extremities" (Cass, 2014). Folic acid (folate) is another B vitamin that helps produce neurotransmitters and hemoglobin, which carry oxygen to the body. Approximately one fourth to one third of depressed people suffer from a folate deficiency. Other symptoms include fatigue, dementia, and problems with the lower extremities (Cass, 2014).

Children who experience constant poor nutrition are at greater risk for mental and emotional health problems, along with psychological disorders that include anxiety and/or learning disabilities. Those children are likely to need mental health counseling, but it's really a diet issue (Fleck, n.d.). Children who suffer from poor nutrition have trouble with proper development and adapting to specific situations, and a link has been revealed by researchers between iron deficiency and childhood hyperactivity disorders (Fleck, n.d.). Bad eating habits, including diets high in sugar and too many skipped meals, have been linked to childhood depression (Fleck, n.d.).

Life Lesson—Candye's Self Esteem

Candye attended my back safety class and was skeptical about my lifestyle advice until she saw my energy level at work. She wrote, "Before attending your class I felt like I was at the end of my rope. I tried all kinds of diets or medications to feel better about myself. My doctor was going to put me on even more medications. I weighed 249 pounds and every day I felt angry, depressed, hungry, irritable, disappointed, fat, ugly, unhealthy, sad, confused, and worthless. I felt like a failure."

Candye explained that she was drinking about seven cans of Mountain Dew every day, eating lots of junk and fried foods, watched TV for hours with no exercise, and had no energy. "I lived to eat. I knew junk food was not good for me, but no one ever explained their horrible consequences on my body until I met you." She was on Zoloft for depression, and had a tubal ligation but was put on birth control pills to control painful menstrual cycles. She took Tylenol with codeine for low back pain, Advil twice a day, blood pressure medicine, and Imitrex for migraines.

Two months after starting my program, she was 30 pounds lighter, wore smaller clothing, stopped drinking soft drinks and eating junk foods, and ate lots of fruits and vegetables. "I have more energy, which has enabled me to cook for my children in the evenings and go for 3-4 mile walks a day. I am not tired all the time and don't require as much sleep as before. I feel happy, excited, positive, focused, healthier and very energetic." Her low back pain was gone, her skin smoother, and her depression and migraines were things of the past. She no longer had pain and abnormal bleeding during her menstrual cycles, which improved her iron deficiency. She noted, "I now eat to live. Everybody deserves to know the facts, as they are, especially those who are in total denial of their poor and irresponsible way of life. Thank you for saving my life."

Praying Over Your Food

Some folks pray over their meals because they're grateful they have something to eat. We've also heard people pray, "Dear Lord, bless this food that we are about to eat for the nourishment of our body and soul, so we can serve you and be an exemplary example to others for your cause." It's a nice prayer, but praying over the indigestible foods on your plate won't suddenly make those foods digestible or great sources of healthy nutrition. For example, both an apple and a hamburger are ingestible substances, but one is digestible and the other is indigestible. Which is which?

You could pray all day over that hamburger and it won't make it digestible, nor will God improve its nutritional quality just because you chose to ingest something unhealthy. But I'll bet you never waste one second praying over the digestible apple. I can thank God for providing me with the apple, but I don't have to ask him to bless the apple because it's already been blessed by God with 10,000 different nutrients—and it will definitely nourish my body based on my experience and experiments I've conducted on myself and my clients over the past 20 years.

Praying for good health can produce good results, but only if it gives us the drive and the motivation to make better choices in life. Otherwise we're living in a fool's paradise, making irresponsible choices, and asking God, the physicians, and other healthcare professionals to fix the mess when the physicians and other healthcare professionals suffer the consequences of their own poor choices.

If your goal is to just manage or control a disease, diseases, conditions, or syndromes, then I suggest you maintain the status quo and continue down the same road you've been traveling. However, the next time you knowingly choose to ingest an indigestible substance, I suggest a different prayer: "Dear Lord, please protect my body from the harmful side effects of this substance I am about to ingest." It's a far more effective prayer.

Chapter 3

Body Chemistry

Normalization of body chemistry begins with diet, not exercise. It is characterized by a body that has a reserve of antioxidants and enzymes from eating a regular diet of raw foods. Raw food consumption minimizes operation of the body's organs and systems, thus allowing them to maintain their vitality and focus on fighting diseases.

Enzymes catalyze food so that cells can be nourished and toxic waste products eliminated. I can't overemphasize that this trio of enzyme functions, nourishment, and waste elimination is the cornerstone of good health. Nourishment and waste elimination are of vital importance in maintaining the body's alkaline chemical balance and preventing obesity.

Enzymes may be divided into two groups: exogenous found in raw foods and endogenous produced within the body. Each of the four enzymes below break down specific components of food—*cellulase* breaks down cellulose, *amylase* breaks down starch, *lipase* breaks down fat, and *protease* breaks down protein. Enzymes are involved in every metabolic activity in the body. They run body organs and systems in a delicate balancing act that determines whether body chemistry is normally slightly alkaline (non-oxidizing) or abnormally acidic (oxidizing).

Enzymes and antioxidants are found and maintained in a healthy, functioning, chemically-balanced immune system that is fueled by raw, uncooked foods. This system defends the body when disease is detected by emitting white blood cells containing enzymes to fight the infection. Antioxidants serve as immune system defense mechanisms that prevent oxidation, a chain reaction caused by the consumption of processed, acidified foods.

An enzyme-depleted immune system has very few defenses (white cells or antioxidants). Without a defense system, processed food puts the body's chemistry in an acidic, oxidizing, diseased state characterized by the presence of charged free radicals, ions, and accumulated cellular waste. Antioxidants, if available, safely interact with free radicals and ions to neutralize them. They return the body chemistry to alkaline by taking electrons from, or donating electrons to, the free radicals or by sharing electrons. Metaphorically speaking, antioxidants are the body's rust inhibitors.

Enzymes also help identify, locate, and isolate disease(s) within the body. Research has shown that the white blood cells contain eight distinctly different *amylase* enzymes. Consequently, there is a direct correlation between the strength of the immune system and the body's enzyme level.

Raw foods supply enzymes and antioxidants that reflect the strength of the immune system, the ability to neutralize free radicals and fight disease, and the amount of energy available to function in work and play, assist in digestion, and minimize stress on organs. They also supply a multitude of organic acids like citric and ascorbic acid that supply an added bonus. Those acids behave like chelating agents that remove and sweep oxidized fat deposits from artery walls. Raw foods prevent and reverse heart disease, high blood pressure, high cholesterol, and diabetes by keeping the body's chemistry slightly alkaline. (See Coronary Heart Disease chapter for details on antioxidants and chelation.)

pH Control

Ross Bridgeford, author of *Alkaline Diet Recipe Book-Vol. 2* (2012), believes there are 12 reasons to avoid acids and keep the body in an alkaline state. Acidic foods make us fat because the body creates fat cells to protect organs from all those excess acids. When the body is totally rid of all acid wastes via a raw diet, it will let them go, which accounts for weight loss experienced when eating raw fruits and vegetables. Further, over acidity of the body reduces our energy levels, increases allergies, and causes damage from free radicals, which leads to premature aging (Bridgeford, 2012). A diet of raw fruits and vegetables also cleanses the body of yeast and fungus overgrowth, which thrive in acidic environments and bring about cravings for more simple sugars. Higher carbohydrate intake also leads to the production of more fat cells, which starts or continues the cycle all over again.

The pH level (the acid-alkaline measurement) of our internal fluids affects every cell in our bodies just like it affects the quality of water in a swimming pool. Extended acid imbalances of any kind create the conditions for obesity, high blood pressure, high blood sugar, high triglycerides, and other diet-related diseases. Metabolic nourishment and elimination processes depend on a balanced, internal alkaline environment. A chronically oxidized, over-acidic pH corrodes body tissue just like it corrodes metal objects exposed to the elements. It slowly eats away at organs, tissues, and 60,000 miles of veins and arteries. If left unchecked, it will interrupt all cellular activities and body functions from the beating of your heart to the air you breathe (Bridgeford, 2012).

People enter the world with a limited amount of enzyme energy that is supplemented and strengthened by mother's breast milk. It's like a bank account. Without regular deposits of exogenous enzymes found in raw foods, body chemistry becomes more acidic. Acid supplies oxygen, leading to the production of charged ions and free radicals that attack the body's veins, organs, and tissues. Acidic, oxidizing chemistry is a dangerous condition that does not manifest itself in obvious ways. It's an insidious, silent killer. Those oxidized species create initiating events that lay the foundation for disease, which I will cover later.

A diet rich in acid-forming food will cause the body to become oxidized, but the majority of people don't know which foods are acid-forming. Sadly, they are frequently found in the typical American diet. Minimizing acid-producing foods and eating a diet high in raw fruits and vegetables cures this. Eating the plantarian way buffers the acid and returns it to a more natural, less reactive, chemically balanced, alkaline state.

A person can live for many years eating processed, enzyme and antioxidant-diminished foods, but this type of diet overworks the body's organs and systems to make up for the shortfall. Eventually, this weakens the immune system and compromises the body's ability to fight diseases. In this condition, arteries begin to clog from oxidized cholesterol, blood pressure rises, and blood sugar increases. Blood sugar continu es to rise because fat cells block pancreatic insulin from metabolizing sugar. Those conditions lead to specific disease-related conditions that attack select organs and systems. For example, when one becomes a Type II diabetic, the heart and kidneys begin to fail, resulting in one or more organs or systems coming under attack or dying every few years. This can lead to loss of vision, limbs, other body parts, or other organ functions.

The ideal way to end life would be for all the body's organs and systems to shut down simultaneously, such as a car battery instead of a flashlight battery that gets weaker and weaker and then dies. A car-battery type of ending is the result of a plantarian lifestyle. Most food-related diseases begin reversing as soon as raw food is introduced to the body. A raw food lifestyle restores the acid-alkalinity balance of the body. In most cases, where disease is diet-related, the need for medication and its side effects can be eliminated. So enzymes in raw, natural foods are of paramount importance to wellness.

Implications for Oxidation and Free Radical Generation

Enzymes maintain the body's alkaline balance. Without supporting that system by consuming exogenous raw food enzymes, the body's normal chemistry changes from alkaline to acidic by oxidizing.

Oxidation creates radicals (often referred to as free radicals), an atomic or molecular species with unpaired (electrically unbalanced) electrons in their outermost ring. Those unpaired electrons are usually highly reactive and seek electrical neutrality by taking electrons from, donating electrons to, or sharing electrons with other atoms. Radicals willingly take part in chemical reactions as a means of seeking electrical neutrality. In the process of seeking neutrality, these highly reactive radicals can cause localized changes to neighboring atoms and molecules by starting a chain reaction. A single charged free radical could cause damage to millions of cells in your body if not neutralized by antioxidants. These pillaging actions build the foundation for unbalanced body chemistry, high blood pressure, high blood sugar, high triglycerides, and a downward health spiral.

Life Lesson—Randy Tells All

Randy was the Safety Supervisor for a local energy company who, along with his co-workers, attended my back safety class, which included the care and nutrition needed to maintain a healthy back (and a healthy total body). The program was adopted by the energy company for their "at risk" employees. Randy wrote, "While the program still explains the mechanics of lifting, the presentations on proper nutrition and stretching add new dimensions to what has otherwise become a passé and trite subject. Our employees have been especially appreciative of the fact that we seem to be genuinely interested in their well-being as opposed to presenting the same old, tired material in a familiar format." I had many opportunities to meet employees of the company in the field and experience the types of work they were doing. It allowed me to personalize my presentation. Randy mentioned that one employee "has gone so far as to tell me that since attending the class, he has embraced the diet changes and has gone from using insulin four times a day over the last twenty years to treat his diabetes, to not having used insulin in the last two months – much to the amazement of his personal physician." Randy also wrote, "The employees who alter their eating and exercise habits will benefit with improved health and longevity."

Those Nasty Free Radicals

Free radical damage to a body is prevented by the body's reserve of antioxidants that neutralize free radicals and terminate the chain reaction before vital cells are damaged. The principle raw food micronutrient (vitamin) antioxidants are vitamin E, beta-carotene, and vitamin C, which are supplied only from raw food and not synthetic vitamin supplements. Additionally, selenium, a trace metal that is required for proper function of one of the body's antioxidant enzyme systems, is sometimes included in this category. The body cannot manufacture those micronutrients so they must be supplied in the diet. A weak, depleted immune system has used up all its antioxidants because they have not been replenished with antioxidant-rich, raw foods such as the ones below.

- Vitamin E, or *d-alpha tocopherol*, is a fat-soluble vitamin present in fresh raw vegetables and fruits, especially apricots and sprouts.
- Vitamin C, or ascorbic acid, is a water-soluble vitamin present in broccoli, cabbage, cantaloupe, citrus fruits, green peppers, kale, kiwi, spinach and strawberries.
- Beta-carotene, a precursor to vitamin A *(retinol)*, is present in broccoli, cantaloupes, carrots, peaches, spinach, squash, tomatoes and sweet potatoes. Because beta-carotene is converted to vitamin A by the body, there is no set requirement. (NOTE: Vitamin A has no antioxidant properties, but can be quite toxic when taken in excess as a vitamin supplement.)

A Note on Detoxification

When dealing with body chemistry, there is no way to avoid discussing detoxification, which is what happens when you change to a diet rich in raw fruits and vegetables. Internally, the human body produces toxins via normal everyday body functions wherein specific biochemical, cellular, and other activities bodily manufacture materials that must be eliminated. When biochemical materials are not eliminated from the body, they can irritate or inflame cells and tissues, block normal cell and organ functions, and even inflame the whole body (Haas, 2005-2014). Toxicity can be caused by drugs that come with side effects, recreational drugs, as well as negative and/or stressful mindsets, toxic foods, alcohol, and emotions that upset the proper functioning of the body (Haas, 2005-2014). Toxicity takes place when the body takes in more than it needs or can use and doesn't eliminate properly.

Some toxins are taken in regularly and in large amounts, and some, such as pesticides and some drugs, do produce immediate symptoms that cause long-term damage. If the body is in a state of optimum wellness, immune functions and the ability to eliminate toxins will work well; but if the body is not in a state of homeostasis, or optimum balance and wellness, toxins will continue to build until the symptoms of illnesses and conditions that may even be life threatening can no longer be ignored. A diet of raw fruits and vegetables can produce the homeostasis we need to achieve optimum wellness.

Chapter 4

Poor Lifestyle Choices & Body Chemistry

Coronary Artery Disease and Cholesterol

High blood pressure injures blood vessel and artery walls. Understanding how the initial injury occurs requires going back to the beginning, when blood flowed unrestricted over electrically neutral vein and artery surfaces. Sometime during this finite period of unrestricted flow, lipid peroxidation (degradation of lipids by free radicals, leading to cell damage) caused by a chemically unbalanced acidic body brought about a change to the electro-chemical potential of a previously electrically neutral deposit site. The difference in electrical potential at the site supplies an attractive force that initiates the deposit of oxidized blood triglycerides and cholesterol. The deposits block blood from getting to the heart, which must exert greater effort to circulate blood throughout the body. This causes high blood pressure, an enlarged, weakened heart, and heart attacks. It also causes the area directly underneath the deposit to exhibit a dangerous chemical imbalance between itself and surrounding tissue that can lead to wall penetration and loss of blood flow.

Cholesterol comes from two places: animal fats in the diet and the liver, which manufacturers it from fat. Therefore, not all cholesterol is bad. Good cholesterol aids in the production of testosterone and estrogen. It is also essential in repairing cell damage due to the presence of free radicals. The liver metabolizes cholesterol by converting it into bile acids used to digest fat. A high-soluble fiber diet absorbs bile acids for secretion from the body. The removal of absorbed bile from the body forces the liver to continually remove cholesterol to sustain bile production. A diet of predominantly processed food causes the liver to recycle used bile acids. The liver subsequently stops absorbing cholesterol to produce new bile acid and cholesterol builds up.

Genetics determine the number of receptors the liver has to metabolize cholesterol. Lifestyle factors also influence the receptor population. Large intakes of dietary fat and cholesterol saturate the receptors and, in doing so, reduce their numbers, which ultimately ends in liver failure. Cholesterol removal is directly proportional to the number of receptors present in the liver. If someone possesses a limited number of receptors and consumes little cholesterol, blood cholesterol stays low. A low number of receptors and a diet high in cholesterol equates to high blood cholesterol levels, high blood sugar, high triglycerides, and high blood pressure.

The total cholesterol level is comprised of two components: LDL (low density lipoprotein) and HDL (high density lipoprotein), or bad cholesterol and good cholesterol. The purpose of HDL is to scavenge LDL and remove excess cholesterol from the bloodstream. A diet of predominantly raw fruits, vegetables, sprouts, and fresh, raw, un-dried nuts will preclude cholesterol from entering the bloodstream and remove any that has accumulated.

Heart Disease

It was once thought that heart disease began in men and women approaching middle or old age. Now we know it sometimes originates in childhood (Story, 2013). The severity of this life-long process is determined early by dietary habits and, to a lesser extent, by physical activity. Today, the symptoms of heart disease actually start in men and women at a very young age. By age twenty-one, many individuals suffer from early onset heart disease.

Many people fail to recognize that heart disease can often be prevented. The Standard American Diet (SAD) of cooked saturated fats and simple carbohydrates abounds at home and in schools, so it's no wonder young people suffer. I think parents and guardians should provide the majority of food for their children by growing it in backyard gardens and orchards. The transformation to manufactured, processed, packaged foods distances us from nature and undermines the body's vitality at an early age.

Parents serve as role models for food choices, and studies show that heart disease is linked to parental influence from birth. At least one in every three children or adolescents experiences obesity, and 90 percent of overweight kids acquire at least one preventable risk factor for coronary artery disease. This means that a significant percentage of our children age prematurely and exhibit "adult" diseases such as high blood pressure and cholesterol. Obese children get bullied a lot, an issue that often surfaces in the news (Teasing, 2013). Eighty percent become obese adults. By the time our children reach their twenties, they are on an established path that leads to coronary-related illnesses and, ultimately, an early death.

While genetics may potentially play a small role, it doesn't account for the huge increase in rates over the past few decades. Genetics can load the gun, but lifestyle choices pull the trigger. To stem the tide of diet-related diseases, we must change the behavioral lifestyles of our children. That starts with changing our own lifestyles to set a positive example for children to mimic. By educating children, serving as role models, and selectively replacing processed foods with proper foods, the incidences of premature, diet-related illnesses and deaths would decline dramatically. Without serious intervention, the current generation of children might be the first in American history to suffer serious illnesses and live shorter lives than their parents. I have witnessed many parents grieving the loss of their children to heart attacks and other diet-related diseases, and I don't believe there is a greater loss or pain for a loving parent than losing a child at any age.

Remember that physical fitness doesn't protect anyone from chronic diseases. For example, great athletes are not afflicted by obesity. Marathoner Jim Fix, who started the running craze, collapsed and died at age 52, at the height of his career and in peak fitness. However, despite his leanness, cholesterol deposits clogged his arteries (Gross, 1984). Grace Kelly's brother, John Kelly, was an Olympic rower and lifelong fitness devotee. After completing a rigorous rowing workout at the Philadelphia Athletic Club, he collapsed and died just outside the club as a result of coronary artery blockage (Goldaper, 1985). Forty-year-old retired basketball legend Pete Maravich collapsed in the midst of a pickup game at a church gym in Pasadena, California, on Jan. 5, 1988, and died from an undiagnosed heart condition (clogged arteries) (Dwyre, 2013).

Health starts on the inside, but people ignore this. Well, I want to right this wrong. I want to scream from the rooftops, "It's not exercise, it's diet!" No matter how fit children become, without a behavioral lifestyle change that restricts processed foods, dietary saturated fats, and simple carbohydrates, heart disease awaits.

Life Lesson—Penny's Story

Penny was admitted to the hospital in September, 2000, for hip replacement surgery, and I was her physical therapist assistant. She attended one of my back safety presentations and she wrote, "In your presentation, not only did you impress me with your knowledge, but also your class was unlike any other class I had ever attended. There are many advocates of healthy living, but very few examples. It was very clear to me that you practice what you teach. The whole presentation kept me on the edge of my seat, wanting to know more."

Penny lost 60 pounds and was able to walk five laps around the mall after working all day. The change of lifestyle has enabled her to stop taking several medications: Verapimil 240mg/day for high blood pressure, half of her Propanolnol dosage, her other blood pressure medicine, Celebrex 600mg daily for arthritis, and Percodan for occasional pain. In her letter, she noted the connection between her high blood pressure and her weight, which she realized was due to her poor eating habits, sedentary lifestyle, and limited physical abilities.

"I have become very active with my children and my grandchildren, have gone from sad to happy, have a new and improved outlook on life, and have applied for a more rewarding job with the state. I could have never accomplished this in my former condition. There are a great majority of people who don't know how to be healthy and the consequences of poor lifestyle choices. I believe you have the ability to change thousands of lives with your program and dedication."

Obesity Again

As stated previously, obesity is not a genetically inherited trait. Obesity starts early in life as a result of parental and other environmental influences that cause the diet to be addictive—rich in saturated fats and processed sugar that unbalance and oxidize the body's chemistry. To a lesser extent, some individuals suffer obesity when, for some reason, the protein leptin fails to send the message that fat cells are full and/or the hypothalamus is unable to read and respond by stopping opioid-induced food craving. The reason for this is currently unknown.

Leptin research on brain feedback is not yet complete, but there are some things we do know (Banks, 2008). A fat cell is capable of storing 1,000 times its initial volume. Each gram of fat contains nine calories. That's a lot when compared with raw proteins and carbohydrates, which have four calories per gram. A person can physically and physiologically consume twice as much raw protein and complex carbohydrates and half as many calories, significantly improving health and reducing excess weight, or even maintaining current weight. Exclusively consuming processed food causes the hypothalamus to recognize the enzyme depletion and then stimulate the body to overeat (Banks, 2008).

Type II Diabetes

Type II Diabetes is a preventable, diet-related disease. Unbalanced body chemistry full of acidic components results from eating processed simple carbohydrates, saturated animal fat, and trans-fats. The insulin secreted by the pancreas will be absorbed by excess fat in the blood that also modifies the shape of the insulin receptor sites located on the cell walls. This slows or prevents recognition of the insulin molecule. Therefore, fat absorption prevents the metabolism of sugar in the body's cells for stabilization. Subsequently, blood sugar levels rise, leading to years of emotional trauma, physical complications, and premature death if not reversed with diet alone.

It is important to remember that medicating to treat any disease will only delay the inevitable. The body will continue to suffer gradually from the degenerative processes created by the medication and the disease itself. Preventing diabetes as well as reversing it is a dual function. It involves reducing the amount of processed food and simple carbohydrates in the diet and increasing the amount of fiber intake from complex carbohydrates. Insoluble fiber from complex carbohydrates promotes slow absorption of sugar, which keeps blood sugar stabilized. Simple carbohydrate sugars are rapidly absorbed in the bloodstream, giving rise to high levels of sugar that cause the all-too-familiar "crash and burn" effect from loading the body with too many simple carbohydrates (Hughes, 2011).

Excess insulin secretion generated to cope with sugar in the blood becomes a double-edged sword. It stimulates the secretion of the enzyme lipase, which absorbs fat from the bloodstream and deposits it in fat cells. Continued exposure to high insulin levels in the blood promotes abnormal growth of cancer and other destructive cells and thickens the arterial muscle (walls), therefore narrowing the arteries. Blood pressure increases, the body gains weight, and is then sucked into a vicious cycle.

It's time to get off the merry-go-round of processed foods, saturated fats, dangerous carbohydrates, fad diets, medications, diet pills, and other don't-work fads. It's time to eat right. As the old, overused expression goes, it's time to *"eat it raw."*

Chapter 5

Through the Age Groups

There's a surplus of information in books and on the internet regarding statistics on age-related illnesses and syndromes. Some discussions include genetic factors, others don't. Some discuss diet, medications, and supplements. Few, if any, discuss ways to prevent those illnesses and conditions. In fact, Internet searches on age-related diseases and illnesses tend to focus on senior citizens and leave other age groups out of the search.

The general consensus on age groupings and health issues starts with birth through 14 years of age. After the age of 14, most children stop seeing a pediatrician and move on to a general practitioner or an internist. The next age groups are 15-30, followed by 30-55, and ending with 55 through the senior-citizen years. However, regardless of the age group, typical illnesses affecting all age groups include occasional colds, flu, pneumonia, other viruses, diarrhea, and urinary tract infections. Conditions and syndromes include, but are not limited to, appendicitis, hernias, kidney stones, hemorrhoids, constipation, allergies, asthmas, headaches, snoring, weight gain, irritability, decreased energy, insomnia, and depression. We are told that such things are normal or routine, but are they? Wasn't the human body created to withstand such an onslaught of illnesses?

As the body ages and people move into their adult years, additional illnesses and conditions include cancer, kidney stones, joint pain, low-back pain, fainting, migraines, gallbladder/digestive diseases, high blood pressure, obesity, high cholesterol/triglycerides, high or low blood sugar levels, heart arrhythmias and other heart-related diseases or syndromes, sleep apnea, hemorrhoids, arthritis, and sleep disorders. Many of those same illnesses or conditions continue as the patient ages and moves into the 55 through senior-citizen years age grouping.

A report from the Centers for Disease Control (CDC) indicates that the general health of Americans hasn't improved very much—six out of every 10 people are either overweight or obese, many still smoke and drink heavily, and many eat poorly. This means that Americans still make lifestyle choices that lead to the high incidence of heart disease, diabetes, and other unremitting illnesses (Thompson, 2013).

The 2013 CDC Report on health in the United States revealed that in 2010, life expectancy at birth for the entire population was 78.7 years, for males it was 76.2 years, and for females it was 81.0 years (Health, 2013). Between 2000 and 2010, life expectancy at birth increased more for the black population than the white population, and during the same time span the infant mortality rate decreased 11 percent—from 6.91 deaths per 1,000 live births to 6.15 (Health, 2013).

The CDC study also revealed that during the same ten-year period, the age-adjusted death rate from heart disease decreased 30 percent—from 257.6 to 179.1 deaths per 100,000—which indicates that 24% of all deaths in the United States were caused by heart disease (Health, 2013). Finally, during the 2000-2010 period, the age-adjusted cancer death rate decreased 13 percent—from 199.6 to 172.8 deaths per 100,000—which indicates that 23% of all deaths in the United States were caused by cancer (Health, 2013). With such improvements reported by the CDC, why is it that Americans are still largely unhealthy? Dr. Linda Mundorff claims that the eating habits of Americans and our inclination to eat unhealthy foods is partly an economics issue—raw produce and other fresh foods are the first to be kicked off the meal-time menu. Time constraints due to working full days and traveling to and from work take away the desire to cook healthy meals. Sometimes healthy foods just aren't available in certain locations and it's cheaper to eat fast food than healthy foods (Murdorff, 2014). As a result, Americans in their middle years may suffer from drug dependency (illegal or legal) and the side effects of those drugs, degenerative joint/disc disease, sluggishness, insomnia, low energy levels, low blood sugar and hypertension, dietary and physical limitations. This is no way to progress through life—a life that should be lived in a healthy and abundant manner. If this is what middle age has become, what is the next age grouping likely to experience? Cancer, with all the accompanying side effects from medications, chemotherapy, and radiation, is one of the top killers of Americans. Heart disease is right up there with cancer, as are strokes, diabetes, and complications from Alzheimer's disease. Those conditions, which don't have to happen, lead to functional and dietary limitations, severe drug dependencies and side effects, depression, dependence on family or outside agencies, placement in a nursing facility or hospice, and eventually death. That is no way to live out the remainder of one's life when it could be prevented.

Life Lesson—Charles & Back Surgery

Charles was a hospital patient whom I encouraged to get out of bed after his serious back surgery. At least that's what he wrote in his letter. He went on to state, "That might seem like a small accomplishment to many, but, considering the serious back surgery I faced, it was a major achievement for me. I also found your discussion of nutrition to be very inspirational." I don't know if Charles followed my suggestions about nutrition, but I doubt he wanted to experience another lengthy hospital stay when it could be prevented.

Ticking Time Clocks

Treatments for all of the illnesses and conditions discussed herein start slowly. Children who do not suffer from chronic or congenital illnesses usually see the doctor for annual check-ups, which include government-mandated vaccines loaded with toxins that have actually done more harm than good, notwithstanding obligatory reports to the contrary (Child, 2010). However, as we age, those visits increase, as do prescriptions for medications and supplements, prescribed exercise and fitness programs, suggested diets, and even surgical procedures.

By middle age, we're in for some serious medical experiences such as joint replacements, a plethora of surgeries, hospitalizations, and an increase in prescribed medications and/or supplements. Our medicine cabinets are filled to overflowing, but we're not getting any better. All we're doing is prolonging the inevitable end and putting toxic Band-Aids on wounds that are still festering, but in most cases will never heal.

According to neuroanthropologist Daniel Lende, the health system in the United States is totally bifurcated, with the top end providing extremely expensive treatments and technologies while the low end receives little or no preventive health care and primary care, and relies almost completely on visits to the emergency room (2012). In truth, neither end is receiving preventative care via diet or any other methodology. Perhaps this is why Lende believes that "[m]edical errors and over-diagnosis and over-treatment can actually drive health problems within the health care system itself" (2012).

For example, the list of *Chronic Disease Statistics* put out by The Center for Managing Chronic Diseases at the University of Michigan revealed the number of Americans, both young and old, who are affected by asthma. Per that list, 9.5 percent (7.1 million) of American children 5-17 years old suffer from asthma that led to 10.5 million days of school missed in 2008 and 754,000 emergency room visits in 2004 (2011). That same list revealed that within the adult population, 8.2 percent (18.9 million) of adults suffer from asthma, which translated into 1.8 million visits to the emergency room in 2004 (2011).

No wonder the healthcare system loves sick people. They and/or their insurance companies are keeping healthcare professionals busy and prosperous. Health care costs Americans more per person than all other nations—including the costs of medicines, medical imaging scans, surgeries, blood analysis, chemotherapy and stays in the hospital—but we have the most totally diseased population (Adams, 2010). The problem isn't the United States; the problem is mainstream medicine that has become a "monopoly medical racket" in this nation for approximately 100 years thanks to enforcement by the Food and Drug Administration (FDA), the American Medical Association (AMA), Federal Trade Commission (FTC), and medical boards in all 50 states (Adams, 2010).

This nation used to be home to fairly healthy people until the medical oligarchy turned it into "a disease dystopia where patients are actually taught that nutrition doesn't work and that they must submit to patented chemicals in order to be 'normal' or healthy" (Adams, 2010). Do you really want to place your health care in the hands of a medical monopoly that chases after high profits at the expense of those it's supposed to be helping? Perhaps this explains why mainstream medicine in the United States has become a corporate endeavor that allows the industry to "claim intellectual ownership over nearly 20 percent of the human genome" (Adams, 2010). That means the medical profession now owns human genes as well as isolated chemicals that were stolen from nature (Adams, 2010). If mainstream medicine were truly effective, doctors wouldn't shy away from natural remedies and proper diets to help their patients get well and/or prevent them from getting sick in the first place. Like the car mechanic who needs sick cars to stay in business, doctors need sick patients to keep their practices up and running at a high profit margin.

Is sound nutrition a good idea? Most Americans would applaud such a concept, but according to the Barna Group, children don't like to eat their vegetables and neither do adults—approximately 63 percent reported they do not eat enough fresh produce and 29 percent of Millennials are seven times more likely than the elderly to express concern about their lack of fruit and vegetable consumption (2014).

This brings us to statistics on one of the epidemics affecting Americans. Diabetes is an epidemic that does severe physical damage, destroys lives, and is killing Americans in all age ranges. The Center for Managing Chronic Disease at the University of Michigan revealed that 25.8 million Americans have diabetes, seven million have the disease but have not been diagnosed, and in 2010 there were 1.9 million new cases in individuals who are age 20 or older (2011).

There were 69,071 deaths cause by diabetes in the United States. 11.9 percent of adults who are age 20 or older have either diagnosed or undiagnosed diabetes, and 8.5 percent of adults in that same age range are definitively diagnosed. Of medical visits, 37.3 million have diabetes as the main diagnosis. Finally, 24 percent of residents in nursing homes are affected with diabetes (Chronic, 2011). Diabetes is not just killing people physically; it is costly to all Americans—the estimated total annual cost is $174 billion (Chronic, 2011).

Finally, the major killer in America before cancer is heart disease, which affects members of all ethnic groups. The CDC reported that approximately 600,000 people die of heart disease in the U.S. every year, which is 25 percent of all deaths (Heart, 2014). It is the main cause of death for men and women, though men were more than half of all deaths due to heart disease in 2009. Coronary heart disease, which is the most common form, kills approximately 380,000 people each year, though approximately 720,000 Americans have heart attacks—515,000 are first heart attacks and 205,000 are repeat attacks (Heart, 2014). The cost to America is approximately $108.9 billion each year, which includes health care, medications, and loss of productivity (Heart, 2014).

Americans are paying out millions of dollars in medical costs and remaining unhealthy—in many instances by choice. They may talk a good game when it comes to taking care of their health, but they rarely "walk the walk" or look for ways to prevent the onset of illnesses in the first place. All they want are magic bullets to fix every health issue rather than taking responsibility for their own physical well-being - and the medical profession is doing nothing to help. In fact, the most significant advances in fighting diseases over the last two centuries were traced to better food, clean drinking water, improved sanitation, better living conditions, and less overcrowding (Child, 2010). Today, diet has become a primary area that goes largely ignored while illnesses, diseases, and even chronic conditions that don't have to occur take their toll on American lives and the lives of millions around the world. The statistics speak for themselves and point to a dismal display of medical guesswork when prevention should be the primary goal.

Chapter 6

Nutrient Myths & Fairy Tales

We are inundated with messages via the internet and media about the importance of nutrients in our foods. One year we hear that something is bad for our health and a decade later the health mavens inform us that the research was wrong, the results were skewed, and the information we were given is false. Perhaps we would fare better if we looked at some of those myths that have permeated the airwaves, magazine and newspaper articles, and even medical journals to get to the truth.

Canola, olive, and safflower oils are healthy

When dealing with oils, we must remember that olive oil comes from olives and safflower oil comes from safflower seeds. The same is true for sesame oil. Yes, it comes from sesame seeds. Assuming a normal processing without chemicals, the oils would not be overtly harmful, though our bodies don't need them. There are no extracted oils that contribute to good health.

However, what about canola oil? We've had it drummed into our heads by doctors, nutritionists, dieticians, and even the media that cooking with canola oil is better for our health. Here's the truth: canola oil is not what you think it is. Canola oil is actually made from the rapeseed, a member of the mustard family, and was originally known as LEAR (Low Erucic Acid Rapeseed), a name which would not appeal to consumers. The name was changed to canola, that is a blend of "Canadian oil" (Axe, 2014). It is industrial oil, not a food, which has been used to produce candles, soaps, lipsticks, lubricants, inks and bio-fuels. In its mixed and genetically modified form, it can cause serious health issues even though it's sold as the best thing since sliced bread because it's low in saturated fats and contains omega-3 fatty acids (Axe, 2014). However, reports on the Internet reveal that canola oil has caused liver, kidney, and even neurological health issues just as health issues arise from genetically engineered corn and soy.

Rapeseed Oil contains high levels of erucic acid, which can cause heart damage. When food manufacturers genetically modified the rapeseed by seed splitting in the 1970s, the result was less erucic acid and higher amounts of oleic acid, which also creates health issues such as abnormal blood platelets, normal growth retardation, damage from free radicals, and elevated risks of cancer (Axe, 2014). Further, the FDA never mentions that aged oils and their exposure to extreme heat for cooking purposes alter their chemical characteristics and renders them more toxic and damaging to the body (High, 2014).

Eating too many fruits causes an undesirable spike in blood sugar

In my practice as a physical therapist assistant, I have never witnessed an abnormal rise in blood sugar by consuming large amounts of fruits. In fact, many with Type II Diabetes benefited from a decrease in the need for insulin (Med, 2008). If humans consumed more fruits and vegetables, they would never develop Type II Diabetes. Further, the likelihood of an expectant mother exhausting her unborn baby's pancreas, which sets the stage for Type I Diabetes—juvenile diabetes would be highly unlikely. This is also true for most other diseases or illnesses.

People with Type I Diabetes also benefit from consuming large amounts of raw fruits and vegetables, and avoiding high animal fat and processed foods. Raw produce decreases the need for insulin because natural sugar is released in a slow and timely manner, which does not overwhelm the digestive system. High animal fat consumption alters the shape of the insulin receptor sites on the cell wall. The result is the inability of cells to recognize insulin molecules, therefore delaying blood sugar storage in the cells. This action prompts the pancreas to produce more insulin, or in the case of the Type I diabetic, prompts more insulin injection. A chronic surplus of insulin is highly detrimental to the health of the vascular system (Diabetes, 2008).

Life Lesson—Maxine Got the Message

Maxine (Max) met me at the hospital where I was working at the time. She wrote, "I have read your material and will speak with my boss and our workers' comp carrier about a pilot project at our facility in Trenton. By the way, I have plenty of fruits and vegetables [and] am hoping this will shock my body and get rid of that last 15 pounds." They say the last 10-20 pounds are the hardest to lose. I disagree. I think they can be lost using a plantarian diet, especially when the body is taking in pure nutrients and eliminating waste in a timely manner

Whole wheat, whole grain, or stone ground bread is healthy

True whole wheat is not genetically modified and grows in fields unmolested. It also doesn't arrive on this planet as sliced bread in plastic bags. When I studied the ingredients in a few brands of whole wheat breads, I noted additives like brown sugar, sugar, molasses, and wheat gluten, all of which harm the body. Wheat consumption alone can harm the body, but soybean oil added to bread is a major source of Omega-6 fatty acid that contributes to poor neurodevelopment in the brain (Gunners, 2014). Omega-3 fatty acid is essential for healthy brain function and is plentiful in raw fruits and vegetables. Unfortunately, many people consume two or three times more Omega-6 than Omega-3, and this consumption is responsible for the degeneration of brain cells. Maybe all that bread is causing brain drains even in those with high intellects.

Consuming dairy products prevents osteoporosis

Dr. Walter Willet is extremely familiar with dairy farming. It's his family heritage. An expert on nutrition at Harvard University, Willet believes that people drink more milk than necessary. He also believes that people don't need to consume dairy products at all and does not see any relationship between dairy consumption and improved bone health (Kirkey, 2014).

Any dairy product manufactured for commercial consumption in America is legally required to use the pasteurization process, which heats the product to destroy bacteria. However, pasteurization destroys the enzymes and the protein necessary for nutrition and metabolism (McAfee, 2012). Dairy products are also potent sources of saturated fat. They tax the digestive system and increase the time food products stay in the bowel, subsequently allowing more time for carcinogens present in the food to mutate into full-blown cancers.

Many children are breast-fed as nature intended. The mother's antibodies are thus transferred to give the child a strong immune system to fight off diseases. A child receives nourishment during the first six months to a year from breast-feeding; after that, he or she is weaned. It is no different in nature. Animals are eventually weaned from their mothers and stop drinking milk. Humans are the only species that continue to drink milk from other animals after weaning, even though the enzymes rennin and lactose required for digesting milk (or any other dairy product) are gone from our systems by age three. Casein from dairy products, though it is needed to build large bones in cows, curdles in the human stomach and tends to line the intestine, thereby hindering the intestines from absorbing nutrients (Myers, 2014).

Meat is a good source of protein, especially if it is lean

Most people love a good meat and potatoes dinner, but is such eating healthy? Meat was a good source of protein when human beings still lived as carnivores in the wild because they didn't want to starve. The digestive systems of carnivores are acid-based, thus aiding in meat digestion. However, the human digestive system is alkaline-based and does not aid in meat digestion. While carnivores break down uric acid found in raw meat with an enzyme called uricase, humans lack this capacity. Since most humans in America live a very modern lifestyle, they do not need to eat meat.

Most humans cook meat, and doing so reduces its nutritional value, destroys all the enzymes, and acidifies the food. Therefore, meat fibers clog the digestive system, add to body toxemia, and make healthy immune systems work overtime. People believe that consuming meat for protein builds bone and muscle, but this is not true. A better source of protein comes from a diet of complex carbohydrates such as raw fruits and vegetables. The complex carbohydrate source of protein keeps the body full of chemistry alkaline, fuels the waste elimination process, and cleanses the body of accumulated toxic material and free radicals (cell waste products). Even "lean protein" clogs and stresses the system (Campbell, 2006).

It gets worse. Protein denatures when it's exposed to a temperature greater than 105.6 degrees. This is why it's dangerous to maintain a body fever of 104 degrees or greater for an extended amount of time—at that point the protein in body cells, especially the brain, literally starts to cook. This creates a condition that may be irreversible and could lead to brain damage. Further, when protein is cooked, the amino acid bonds break up, take on a different form that renders them ineffective as a familiar protein, and could take on a form that may even be more harmful to the body.

So while meat provides a living for gourmet food authors and Cordon Bleu chefs, it results in no quality of life and yields a dividend of illnesses even if eaten in moderate quantities. Yes, it provides short-lived emotional comfort, but the only contribution cooked meats make to the human condition is the supply of a leading source of cholesterol and fat while taxing the digestive system and shortening the human lifespan. How much do you want that hamburger, steak, or barbequed ribs now?

Eat dark chocolate to protect against heart disease

While it sounds like a tasty way to stay healthy, it's important to know that chocolate is a man-made derivative of cocoa beans. When the beans are fresh they contain antioxidants called flavanols that are beneficial to the blood flow and vascular function. In their fresh-picked state, cocoa beans taste bitter, so harmful chemicals, flavorings, and sugar are added to make the chocolate taste good. This process strips the heart-protecting flavanols and other nutrients, and renders the chocolate harmful to the heart and overall health if consumed regularly (Parker-Pope, 2007). My advice is to occasionally enjoy any kind of chocolate for its taste, but not for its healthful properties because there are none. Just don't tell Godiva, Hershey's, or those cute and colorful little M&M guys.

Drink one or two glasses of wine for a healthy heart

It seems that every time the wine industry has a lag in sales, they come up with favorable published studies by a paid scientist to boost sales. And consumers always find a reason to justify irresponsible behavior, including demanding that supermarkets sell wine. Who can blame them? For years nutritionists claimed that a glass of wine each day was good for the circulatory system, but a paper published in the British Medical Journal stated that drinking less decreases the risk of heart disease and lowers blood pressure (Spencer, 2014).

According to Professor Juan Casas at the London School of Hygiene and Tropical Medicine, there is a link between less consumption of alcohol and better cardiovascular health. The study showed that drinking only two glasses of wine each day will harm your health (Spencer, 2014). Add to those findings the scam about resveratrol, a natural phenol manufactured by several plants when they are attacked by bacteria or fungi. It is also found in great quantity in the skin of red grapes and other fruits, but red wine contains very little resveratrol (Isaacs, 2012).

Commercial products containing this much-touted miracle cure, which it is not, are produced using chemical and biological synthesis, and supplements come mainly from Japanese knotweed (Isaacs, 2012). Not only did the wine industry benefit from flawed studies, the supplement industry went haywire producing resveratrol pills, capsules, and tonics for brainwashed consumers who, again, wanted a magic bullet to feel healthy. I don't condone drinking alcohol or any other mind altering drinks because neither contributes anything positive to good health.

Further, consumption of one or two glasses of wine every night to relax before bedtime means you're likely suffering from alcoholism, and the British study did reveal that many participants did not tell the truth about the extent of their alcohol consumption (Spencer, 2014). They also didn't divulge the frequency with which they held a glass of wine in their hands while shouting, "Bottoms up!" Admitting there's a problem is the first step to recovery and reversal of this harmful and irresponsible behavior.

Raw nuts and seeds are great sources of protein

This is true if the nuts or seeds are picked right off the trees or eaten from the inside of the produce. I almost fell off my chair when I heard a cardiologist on TV tell the audience to purchase raw nuts and keep them fresh in the refrigerator. It's just not possible! They're never refrigerated in the stores that sell them; they sit in bins getting stale, dehydrated, moldy, and full of rancid oils. The only healthy nuts are the ones that are freshly picked because they still contain the right amount of water to keep all the nutrients in the seeds alive and healthy.

Then there's the truth about raw nuts that would make the wisest consumer think twice about purchasing them. If those raw nuts haven't been soaked or dried, they can be dangerous because they contain harmful substances and enzymes that stop the plant from sprouting too soon and prevent invasion by hungry insects. Further, without soaking the raw nuts, the phytic acid in them may protect the plant but it can lead to nutrient deficiencies and stop the body from absorbing calcium, magnesium, iron, and zinc (Robin, 2014).

Add to that the bacteria found in raw nuts—raw almonds were the cause of several outbreaks of salmonella. Those almonds were grown in California, the largest almond grower in the U.S. Now, California bans their sale, though blanching, light steaming and heat kill the salmonella, along with some nutrients (Robin, 2014). Peanuts are not innocent bystanders in the raw nuts dilemma, notwithstanding the dancing peanut guy with the cute top hat. They contain aflatoxins that can cause severe illness and roasting only kills approximately 50 percent of those aflatoxins in nuts. However, roasting is not the best solution because chemicals like acrylamide form during the process, and such chemicals are carcinogenic to animals and most likely to humans (Robin, 2014).

Nuts are tasty and make people feel as if they're snacking on something healthy, but they have little to no nutritional value. They just sit in your stomach the way any animal product or cooked substance would, which gives those consuming them a sense of fullness and a false sense of high protein intake. Save your money! Better to feel satiated by foods that really are healthy and packed with nutrients than foods that do nothing for your health and wellness.

Strong food cravings indicate you are deficient in the chemicals found in those foods

The craving for a specific food is the result of taste bud conditioning and memory. Retraining the taste buds to desire more raw fruits and vegetables by eating more raw fruits and vegetables can curb such cravings. Brian Wansink, PhD, director of Cornell University's Food and Brand Lab, studies the relationship people have with food, including food cravings (Kam, 2014). Author of the book *Mindless Eating: Why We Eat More Than We Think*, his goal is to "uncover eating traps and change them" (Kam, 2014).

Wansink believes that understanding food cravings is a must because we are inundated with environmental flags, such as sight or smell, that cause us to eat too much, and the old myth that we crave what our bodies need is just that—a myth. Marcia Pelchat, PhD, researches food at the Monell Chemical Senses Center in Philadelphia, where she has shown that food cravings occur even when a diet is calorically and nutritionally sufficient. However, blaming nutritional needs for the cravings makes us feel less guilty when that craving is nothing more than an obsession about a food we want to eat (Kam, 2014).

While food cravings are considered normal during pregnancy, they occur because of an increase in hormone levels that affects saliva, mirroring the chemical content of the blood and altering the taste of food (Richards, 2011). One study showed that women who ate fruits and vegetables during their pregnancies had babies who became accustomed to the taste of those fruits and vegetables. They were also protected against abnormal growth and possible juvenile diabetes when compared to babies born to mothers who did not eat fruits and vegetables while pregnant (Richards, 2011). You and your baby don't need that bag of potato chips loaded with salt or the box of cookies filled with sugar because you don't need the salt and sugar and neither does your baby.

Juices & smoothies are as good as raw fruits and vegetables

This is a huge myth! The truth is that juicing destroys the harmonious physiological balance among the nutrients, as well as the consistency and integrity of the fiber and other important nutrients in the fruits and vegetables. Drinking fruit juice causes an abnormal spike in blood sugar and forces the pancreas to pump insulin into the blood. Even moderate, but continuous consumption of fruit juices of any kind will harm the health of the vessels. Further, consuming fruit juice or any liquid form of food—either smoothies or nutrient drinks—will stop important interactions with certain digestive enzymes that are imperative in digestion and nutrient absorption because of its short period of residency and exposure in the digestive system.

A normal and healthy digestion process begins with the enzymes in the mouth. These enzymes are activated by chewing food, which then travels down through the esophagus into the stomach. A specific set of enzymes begin to interact with the chewed food as it moves along the digestive tract. Typically the stomach doesn't work very hard to digest a food that is already nutrient dense, such as raw fruits and vegetables. But if it's nutrient depleted junk, processed or cooked, it will have to sit there for a while until the body is able to begin the enzymatic reactions using borrowed vitamins, minerals, and enzymes from the body's reserve. That digested substance is then passed through the small and the large intestines.

Throughout this whole process the ingested substance has continuous close contact with the interlining of our digestive system, which is responsible for the absorption of nutrients and water from the ingested substance. The substance is slowly moved forward in the stomach into the small and large intestines by a smooth muscle action called peristalsis. This action is slow so the body has sufficient time to absorb all the nutrients necessary to fuel and repair the body's cellular system. When food is in the form of liquid only, it will pass through the digestive system very quickly and not afford the body the potential benefits found in food in its whole state.

Add to that the fact that your body doesn't use any energy to break down the juiced "food," meaning calories derived from the natural sugars in the juice aren't balanced by those commonly used in digestion of solid foods (Coleman, 2012). This lack of vitamins and nutrients absorbed by the body will gradually become visible in the way of hair loss, dry skin from lack of fatty acids, eczema if the skin is already dry, premature aging of the skin, damage to the teeth, and a lack of energy (Coleman, 2012).

In my busy lifestyle, I look for the easiest and fastest way to consume my nutrients. Grab an apple and run with it. Apples are the best and fastest "fast food" nature has to offer. Unless you're able to hire someone to clean the juicer or blender every time you use it, or you do not care to have the maximum amount of nutrient absorption for your buck, then juicing and smoothies have your name written all over them. Drink up, but don't expect great results. Expect the opposite.

Vitamin supplements are necessary

Millions of people take vitamin and mineral supplements at a cost of billions of dollars each year, but real vitamins are not found in doctors' offices, bottles on the shelves in drug stores, and not even on the shelves in "health food" stores. They are found in the earth—in the plants, bushes, vines on trees, and orchards around the world.

Supplements constitute a modern-day form of quackery that enriches vitamin companies and their stockholders. Nothing in scientific literature supports the use of supplements, and people should read the disclaimers on bottles before wasting hard-earned money and endangering their health. A label that reads, "This product is not intended to diagnose, treat, cure or prevent any disease" says it all. As long as a person's diet consists of uncooked foods, the body will extract and absorb all of its vitamin needs, metabolize the natural vitamins from food, not be subjected to man-made concoctions with no proven efficacy, and not suffer element imbalances from ingested supplements.

Contrary to popular belief, regular consumption of raw fruits and vegetables does prevent and cure most lifestyle chronic diseases and disorders. There are thousands of unidentified micronutrients that exist in raw foods, and in order for the nutrients to benefit the body, they will have to work in concert with other key nutrients in a nutritionally well-balanced environment. It is ridiculous to think that extracted or synthetic vitamins are able to carry out the same task. Vitamin manufacturers are incapable of mimicking the correct balance of the ingredients that exist in whole fruits and vegetables, and this imperfection can lead to undesirable side effects.

For example, in 1994, the National Cancer Institute collaborated with Finland's National Public Health Institute and studied 29,000 Finnish men over

50 years old who were long-term smokers. All were at high risk for cancer and heart disease and were given either vitamin E or beta-carotene, both, or neither one (Offit, 2013). There was no doubt about the results of the study, though the researchers were surprised. Those taking vitamins and supplements were in far greater danger of dying from lung cancer or heart disease compared to those who didn't take the vitamins (Offit, 2013).

The same results occurred in a 1996 study at the Fred Hutchinson Cancer Research Center in Seattle, Washington, where researchers studied 18,000 people who were at high risk for lung cancer because of exposure to asbestos (Offit, 2013). The subjects were given vitamin A, beta-carotene, both vitamins, or neither one, but the study was stopped immediately when it was determined that those taking the supplements were dying from cancer and heart disease far faster than those who took no supplements (28 percent higher for cancer and 17 percent higher for heart disease) (Offit, 2013).

Want more proof? On October 10, 2011, University of Minnesota researchers studied 39,000 older women who were taking supplemental multivitamins, magnesium, zinc, copper, and iron. Those women died at rates higher than those who didn't (Offit, 2013). Two days later, Cleveland Clinic researchers issued the results of a study of 36,000 men who took vitamin E, selenium, both, or neither supplement and found that taking vitamin E increased the chances of prostate cancer by 17 percent (Offit, 2014).

An article in the October 25, 2011, edition of *The Wall Street Journal* supports what I've been saying about eating raw fruits and vegetables. Josephine Briggs, who heads up the National Center for Complementary and Alternative Medicine (an NIH center), believed that the huge volume of data accrued to date proved that a plant-rich diet is healthy and taking anti-oxidants and other nutrients out and putting them in pills is not consistently beneficial (Wang, 2011). That data and information was discovered by the big guns in medical research. Maybe it's time we paid attention and stopped loading our bodies with vitamins and supplements we don't need or that will harm us in the short and long-run. (See Chapter 18: Why No Supplements? for more information on this issue.)

Read nutrition/food labels

It seems that more and more people read nutrition labels hoping to find the healthiest foods, but their efforts are a waste of time. The truth: If you're reading the food labels, you aren't eating properly. While the Federal government mandated proper food labeling by manufacturers starting in 1990, the nutritional value of food can be fudged by as much as 20 percent and still fall within government guidelines. Further, government food labs have a ten percent margin of error, and there is also a ten percent testing margin of error. So, if a food item label shows 500 calories, it can legally contain as many as 600 calories.

Another very important note: If you are considering calories and other nutritional contents on boxed food, chances are you already suffer from health issues you want to correct. Checking labels is not the way to do it. Food manufacturers are well aware that shoppers are looking to buy healthier foods, so they take every occasion to include health claims on the front label of their products. But those claims don't tell the whole truth, and shoppers don't know which are true and which aren't. That makes food shopping more complicated than it was before all those mandatory labels arrived on grocery shelves.

Food manufacturers don't just use legal loopholes to hide the truth, they literally mislead consumers. For example, "all-natural" applies only to meat and eggs, and means minimal processing and no artificial ingredients. Unfortunately, both may be accurate, but that doesn't mean the ingredients are healthy (Chatsko, 2014). When it comes to "gluten-free" foods, the USDA rules are so confusing that all food manufacturers will capitalize on the confusion. After all, who's going to check on the $5 billion gluten-free industry? (Glatsko, 2014).

"Cage-free" is another misleading claim that tells consumers all those birds were allowed to run around their "homes" and had complete access to food and clean water while they were roaming freely. But broiler chickens, which are raised for meat, are not kept in cages. They are cage-free because that's the way it's always been done (Glatsko, 2014). Ironically, the government says it's not legal to put "antibiotic-free" on food packaging, so manufacturers changed the wording to "raised without antibiotics," a phrase often used during commercials for certain restaurants that goes unchallenged (Glatsko, 2014).

Finally, there's the "raised without hormones" claim, which is absurd since federal regulations have never allowed hormones or steroids to be used in pork, poultry, or goat. Evidently, no one is monitoring this regulation because Horizon organic dairy milk made by WhiteWave Foods has a statement on their products that reads, "No significant difference has been shown between milk from [growth hormone-treated] and non-[growth hormone-treated] cows" (Glatsko, 2014).

If hormones used in cows do not affect humans who consume milk from those cows, why bother with the disclaimer? Those growth hormones have been proven to be harmful to your health to the point that medical groups have demanded the process stops. Recommendations from the American Public Health Association and American Nurses Association, among other medical groups, include denouncing drinking milk that comes from cows that are given "GM bovine growth hormone, because the milk from treated cows has more of the hormone IGF-1 (insulin-like growth factor 1)—which is linked to cancer" (IRT, 2006-2014).

Clearly, you must educate yourself. While you can eat what you want, know that you are largely being misled by those producing most of the foods you consume. You don't need a degree in nutrition to make heads or tails of those labels, you just have to be patient and do the necessary research to find the truth. Conversely, you can stop reading labels on all those foods that won't do you any good and just eat raw fruits and vegetables. And if you happen to be an animal lover, you cannot pick and choose which animal will be spared and which will be eaten. It just doesn't work that way.

Chapter 7

The Tidal Wave of Nutrients

I often ask people why they are afraid or reluctant to move toward a healthier way of living that will produce wellness. Most are locked into their current lifestyles and are concerned the change will be too difficult or even too expensive. The first may be true, depending on your attitude, but the second is totally untrue. Further, there are a myriad of advantages to a plant-based diet, the first of which is no calorie counting. Add to that not having to weigh what you eat or watch food intake levels to either lose weight or maintain a healthy weight. Plant-based diets provide all the nutrients your body needs to maintain good health and wellness.

When examining plant foods and animal foods, it is important to consider their "nutritional totality as a group" in order to understand the differences in their nutrient makeup (Joyful, n.d.). While animal-based foods do have nutritional value, those nutrients do not affect the body positively with regard to chemical and biological effects (Joyful, n.d.).

Foods from the animal food group produce free radicals in our bodies when they are metabolized, but foods that are plant based are full of antioxidants that help cleanse the body of free radicals while providing thousands upon thousands of densely packed nutrients that increase cell functions. This includes high levels of fiber, beta-carotene, and greater amounts of vitamins C, E, and folate. According to T. Colin Campbell, PhD, and Thomas M. Campbell II, authors of *The China Study*, plant foods as a group provide the body all needed nutrients along with protection from diseases (Campbell & Campbell, 2006). The chart below, from TheVeganRoad.com, shows the differences in nutrient composition between plant and animal food groups. Notice that the first item on the chart is cholesterol. There is no cholesterol in a plant-based diet, but there is in animal-based foods. While we do need some cholesterol for our bodies to function properly—support cell membranes and tissues that surround the nerves—the body is capable of making the right amount of cholesterol to handle those functions (Principles, 2014). It is also obvious how much higher the nutrient content is in the plant foods compared to animal foods.

Nutrient Composition of Plant and Animal-Based Foods (per 500 calories of energy)

Nutrient	**Plant-Based Foods***	Animal-Based Foods**
Cholesterol (mg)	—	137
Fat (g)	4	36
Protein (g)	33	34
Beta-Carotene (mcg)	29,919	17
Dietary Fiber (g)	31	—
Vitamin C (mg)	293	4
Folate (mcg)	1,168	19
Vitamin E (mg_ATE)	11	0.5
Iron (mg)	20	2
Magnesium (mg)	548	51
Calcium (mg)	545	252

** Equal parts tomatoes, spinach, lima beans, peas, potatoes.*

*** Equal parts beef, pork, chicken, whole milk.*

Two issues that usually arise are the levels of vitamins B-12 and D. This is a specific concern for the elderly, many of whom suffer from malabsorption issues. However, vitamin D is not really a vitamin because "a vitamin is a nutrient we have to consume because we don't make it" (Principles, 2014). Vitamin D is comprised of many chemicals, with natural vitamin D being produced in the skin from an ever-present type of cholesterol called 7-dehydrocholesterol (Harvard, 2007). The key is sunlight: "the sun's ultraviolet B (UVB) energy changes the precursor to vitamin D3" (Harvard, 2007). In essence, the energy of the sun turns a chemical in the skin into vitamin D-3, which is carried to the liver and then the kidneys to convert it to active vitamin D (Harvard, 2007). That means that all those hours at the pool are helping to load you up with what you need to make vitamin D.

B-12 is another story. While some say vitamin B-12 is only available via meat, eggs, cheese, and other animal sources, it's available in lower amounts through plants via synthesis of microorganisms (Principles, 2014). Plants grown in organic soil filled with microorganisms that haven't been killed off by pesticides are a good source of B-12 (Principles, 2014). This is nothing to ignore.

In today's food supply, the most prevalent source of B-12 is animal products. However, cows do not make B-12, "but the bacteria in its gut does." When cows eat grass, they get B-12 from the enriched soil attached to the grass, which "allows the bacteria in the gut to make use of the B-12 thereby imparting it to the animal" (Knutson, 2014). That's how those who came way before us did well on plant-based foods without adding supplements. Their foods came from the ground and all the soil, rich in B-12, could never fully be removed (Knutson, 2014).

Not so today. Food is cleaned, processed, stored, sold, and cleaned again when we bring it home. The B-12 is being washed down the drain because most of us just don't like to eat dirt. Remember, cooked animal products don't provide us with adequate B-12 or any other essential nutrients. If you're adamant that you have to eat animal products to get your B-12, it can be up to five percent of your overall food intake.

Further, one of the main reasons people are skeptical about eating only a raw plantarian diet is the fear that they won't get enough protein. It is not based on any factual data or research. Animal protein is viewed as a macronutrient that is essential for building muscles and strength. The best way that I can explain the presence of protein in plants is that all plants have to have all the essential and non-essential macro and micronutrients in order to grow to maturity and become fruitful and productive. Protein is one of the essential macronutrients that plays an important role in the plant cell. When we consume raw fruits or vegetables, we ingest that protein and it is processed to build our muscles. Without the presence of protein or any other essential nutrients, the plant will either not grow to maturity or produce mutant fruits that may be distasteful and not be very pleasing to the eyes. If it's still difficult to wrap your head around this, you may want to observe all the muscular grazing animals.

You should also note that calories from fruits and vegetables are nutrient-dense so there is no need to limit certain ones based on the amount of calories present in the produce. Nutrients from raw fruits and vegetables are self-regulated and there is no risk of overdosing or exceeding the recommended daily allowance.

So, let's look at some of the plant-based foods we can eat while enjoying the journey to wellness. I've divided them into two groups, fruits and vegetables, and chosen a sampling from each group. Just remember that each food contains specific nutrients important for overall wellness. Note: be sure to check out

Dr. Decuypere's Nutrient Charts at http://www.health-alternatives.com/fruit-nutrition-chart.html. You'll find charts for fruits and vegetables that will help you create the right plant-based diet mix.

FRUITS

ACEROLA CHERRIES — The U.S. Department of Agriculture (USDA) claims that acerola cherries have the most amount of vitamin C compared to other food sources. In fact, their juice is so rich in vitamin C, it should not be taken with other vitamin C supplements (Busch, 2014). They do not freeze well, have a rapid rate of deterioration (within four hours after harvesting), and fermentation occurs in three to five days, which is why are used in sugary jams, syrups, and juices (Busch, 2014). While I'm not a fan of juicing at all, one cup of fresh (and I mean fresh) acerola juice does provide 1,232 international units of vitamin A, mostly in the form of beta-carotene and half the amount in the fresh berries (Busch, 2014). The freshly picked berries also contain flavonoids, which are a form of antioxidants. However, I do not recommend juicing because of the damaging effects of the high sugar concentration.

APPLES — One medium-size, unpeeled apple provides 0.47 grams of protein, 95 calories, and 4.4 grams of dietary fiber. Apples are a good source of boron, which affects electrical activity in the brain and aids calcium absorption. Boron increases mental alertness and estrogen in postmenopausal women. Apples contain selenium, which is thought to lower the risk of asthma, and are excellent sources of antioxidants. In fact, apples contain over 10,000 nutrients, which may explain the "an apple a day keeps the doctor away" slogan. But a few apples before going to bed makes the doctor beg for his bread. From my own experience of eating several apples a day, I sometimes find this to be more fact than fiction.

Life Lesson—Jill's Pound Cake

She wrote about my "enlightening and amazing presentation," and mentioned that everyone in attendance was "bowled over." I didn't notice the "bowled over" status of all the attendees, but I did get a sense that mental wheels were turning as information was provided to them. Jill wondered "how many of our folks will be seen at a produce stand today buying FRESH veggies and fruit. I know I will!" What more could I ask of such a delightful woman who was smart enough to let me know that "that slice of pound cake y'all saw me with last night landed in the garbage. Instead I munched on the two delicious Cameo apples"—the ones I distributed to all in attendance. Jill found this very symbolic and a way to start them on a program of healthy eating. She also thanked me for my opinion "concerning strenuous exercise" because she was glad to learn that she just needs to "stay active, walk, swim, and do some resistance repetitions." The best testimonial from Jill was tossing out the pound cake and chomping on those apples.

AVOCADOS — One medium-size avocado provides 4.02 grams of protein, 322 calories, and 13.5 grams of fiber. Health benefits of avocados include reduced cholesterol levels, reduced risk of diabetes, help reducing weight, and cancer prevention. Avocados can actually be a complete or near-complete part of any meal. According to a study published in the *Archives of Medical Research*, a diet rich in avocados can improve a person's lipid profile in healthy patients and even in patients with mildly high cholesterol and triglycerides (MNT, 2014). The study revealed that one week after adhering to an avocado-enriched diet, the patients' bad cholesterol and triglycerides levels decreased by 22 percent and good cholesterol increased by 11 percent (MNT, 2014). Another study published in the 2013 issue of the *Nutrition Journal* noted that avocados improved an overall intake of nutrients and reduced the risk of diabetes, stroke, and coronary artery disease (all labeled as metabolic syndromes) (MNT, 2014).

BANANAS — One medium-size banana provides 1.29 grams of protein, 105 calories, and 3.1 grams of dietary fiber. Bananas, which are high in vitamin B-6, aid in weight reduction, decrease swelling, defend against development of Type-2 diabetes, reinforce the nervous system, and aid in the production of white blood cells (Szalay, 2014). Bananas are good for your heart, protect the cardiovascular system, and guard against high blood pressure because they are loaded with potassium. Bananas also contain high levels of magnesium and tryptophan, which is converted to serotonin, a mood elevator (Szalay, 2014). Eaten in moderation, they aid in digestion and weight reduction, help with vision because of their high vitamin A content, help maintain bone health, and protect against kidney cancer (Szalay, 2014).

BLUEBERRIES — One cup of blueberries provides 1.1 grams of protein, 84 calories, and 3.6 grams of dietary fiber. Research has shown that blueberries have the highest concentration of antioxidants when compared with 40 other fresh fruits. Blueberries contain vitamins A and C, zinc, potassium, iron, calcium and magnesium. They are also high in fiber and low in calories (Boulanger, 2013).

CRANBERRIES — One cup of cranberries provides 0.39 grams of protein, 46 calories, and 4.6 grams of dietary fiber, and 8,983 total antioxidant capacity—"wild varieties have 13,427; cultivated cranberries have 9,019" (Davis, 2005-2014). Fresh, uncooked cranberries are rich in polyphenols and are an excellent source of antioxidants. Research has demonstrated that they inhibit the growth of breast cancer cells and reduce the risk of gum disease and stomach ulcers. Fresh, whole berries should not be confused with cranberry juice, which is high in sugar. These berries are delicious in a salad.

ORANGES — One medium-size orange provides 1.23 grams of protein, 62 calories, and 3.1 grams of dietary fiber. Oranges also contain every class of cancer inhibitor known to science, including beta-carotene, terpenes, and flavonoids. They are rich in vitamin C and are thought to defend against asthma, bronchitis, breast and stomach cancer, and gum disease. Oranges lower cholesterol, optimize heart function, lower risk of disease, and help with vision (Coffman, n.d.).

PAPAYAS — One cup of cubed fresh papaya provides 0.85 grams of protein, 55 calories, and 2.5 grams of dietary fiber. This fruit is a concentrated source of boron and papain that contains powerful antioxidants, vitamins C and A, beta-carotene and potassium. Papaya aids digestion, reduces the risk of heart disease, diabetes, and cancer, improves blood glucose levels, lowers blood pressure, and improves wound healing (MNT, 2014).

PEACHES — Not enough can be said for the goodness of peaches. One unpeeled, medium-size peach provides 1.36 grams of protein, 58 calories, and 2.2 grams of dietary fiber. Peaches contain boron, are rich in antioxidants and beta-carotene, and are low in saturated fat, cholesterol, and sodium (Scutti, 2013). They are loaded with 10 different vitamins—A, C, E, K, and six of the B complex vitamins. Vitamin A and beta carotene help with producing optimal vision, while the antioxidant vitamin C helps the immune system.

Peaches are also a good source of folate, pantothenic acid, thiamin, riboflavin, vitamin B-6, niacin, and folate—nutrients needed by all the cells and nerves, as well as fiber (Scutti, 2013). Just as important is the potassium in peaches , which helps reduce the incidence of diseases of the kidneys as well as ulcers. Peaches also contain magnesium, phosphorus, zinc, copper, manganese, iron, and calcium, which protect and support red blood cells, the nervous system, and the bones (Scutti, 2013). The stone fruits, like peaches, contain bioactive compounds that have also been found to reduce metabolic syndromes via phenolic compounds, which have anti-obesity, anti-inflammatory, and anti-diabetic capabilities (Scutti, 2013).

PINEAPPLES — Pineapples are nutrient dense, cholesterol-free, and fat-free. One cup of cubed pineapple contains 80 calories, 2 grams of fiber, 1 gram of protein, 40 percent of your daily need of vitamin C, 10 percent of thiamine, 8 percent of B-6, six percent of magnesium, and four percent of riboflavin, folate, niacin and iron (Bruso, 2014). Pineapple is high in manganese for osteoporosis prevention, and the amount of bromelain present is a protease with some anti-inflammatory and anti-edema properties. This tropical fruit aids in digestion, helps dissolve blood clots, and has anti-bacterial and anti-viral properties. A nutrient-dense food, pineapple helps with weight loss—it makes you feel full by providing fiber, and essential vitamins and minerals without adding too many calories (Bruso, 2014).

RASPBERRIES — One cup of fresh raspberries contains 1.48 grams of protein, 64 calories, and 8 grams dietary fiber in the form of pectin, which is believed to lower cell damage, thus decreasing cholesterol. That same cup of raspberries contains 186 mg of potassium needed to maintain healthy blood pressure, 31 mg of calcium for bone development and growth, and 167 combined mcg of lutein and zeaxanthin (Sarao, 2013). Lutein and zeaxanthin are carotinoids (plant pigments) which help protect against macular degeneration, which can cause loss of vision. In that same one-cup serving is up to 26 mcg of folate, which helps prevent neural tube defects in newborns (Sarao, 2013). Raspberries also contain large amounts of anthocyanins and cancer-fighting agents such as ellagic, coumaric and ferulic acid. They also contain vitamins A, C and E, used to fight inflammatory conditions, e.g., arthritis and gout, by stopping the body's inflammatory response enzymes (Sarao, 2013).

STRAWBERRIES — One cup of whole strawberries contains 0.96 grams of protein, 46 calories, 2.9 grams of dietary fiber, and comes close to blueberries by providing antioxidants thought to prevent the oxidation of cholesterol. One serving also provides 51.5 mg of vitamin C, approximately half of your daily requirement. Strawberries are an outstanding source of folate, a plus for the elderly because inadequate amounts of folate (folic acid) contribute to vascular disease, atherosclerosis, and reduced brain/cognitive function (Daniluk, 2014). Note that medicines prescribed for conditions like rheumatoid arthritis reduce or deplete folic acid, but strawberries can replenish what is lost (Daniluk, 2014). Strawberries show signs of being able to suppress inflammatory responses as well as reduce the risk of hypertension by lowering LDL cholesterol (Daniluk, 2014). Strawberries are also high in potassium, which reduces bone loss by maintaining stores of calcium that prevent the effects of aging on the bones. Strawberries contain anthrocyanin, an antioxidant that provides an excellent defense against free radicals from the environment, including the sun.

WATERMELON — One medium slice of watermelon, which is about two cups of the edible part, contains 1.74 grams of protein, 86 calories, 1.1 grams of dietary fiber, and is high in lycopene, a nutrient important for heart health. Each cup contains 46 calories, 20 percent of your daily intake of vitamin C, 17 percent of vitamin A, and potassium, which regulates blood pressure.

VEGETABLES

BROCCOLI — One half cup of broccoli contains 1.86 grams of protein, 27 calories, 2.6 grams of dietary fiber, and anti-cancer antioxidants such as beta-carotene, vitamin C, and indoles. It contains chromium to help regulate insulin and blood sugar. Broccoli also contains glucoraphanin that the body converts into an anti-cancer compound called sulforaphane which removes H. pylori, a bacterium that tends to raise the risk of [stomach ulcers) and gastric cancer (Herrington, 2012). It also contains indole-3-carbinol, a potent antioxidant complex and anti-carcinogen that stops the growth of breast, cervical, and prostate cancer while boosting liver function. The soluble fiber content is high enough to help remove cholesterol from the body and, as a significant source of anti-inflammatory phyto nutrients kaempferol and isothiocyanates, broccoli lowers the impact of allergy-related substances on the body (Herrington, 2012). It is a significant source of vitamin C and flavanoids, lutein, zeaxanthin and beta-carotene, calcium, and vitamin K. Broccoli can help prevent or reverse damage to the linings of blood vessels due to chronic blood sugar syndromes via the anti-inflammatory abilities of sulforaphane. Broccoli also detoxifies the body due to its high content of special phytonutrients and isothiocyanates, which help the detox process at a genetic level (Herrington, 2012).

CABBAGE — One half cup of cabbage contains 0.95 grams of protein, 17 calories, and 1.4 grams of dietary fiber. There are several varieties of cabbage such as white, purple and green. The purple variety contains anthocyanins, which have been documented as anti-carcinogenic, is extremely low in saturated fat and cholesterol, and is high in fiber, folic acid, vitamin C and vitamin K (Bollacker, 2012). As with other green vegetables, cabbage is an excellent source of riboflavin, pantothenic acid, and thiamin, a natural source of electrolytes and minerals such as calcium, potassium, phosphorous, manganese, iron and magnesium (Bollacker, 2012).

CARROTS — A medium-size carrot has 25 calories, 6 grams of carbs, and 2 grams of fiber. It is an outstanding source of beta-carotene, a natural chemical the body changes into vitamin A. One carrot provides over 200 percent of the daily requirementof beta-carotene and the deeper the orange color, the higher the beta-carotene content (Thompson, 2005-2014). Carrots are powerful cancer fighters, artery protectors, immune boosters, and contain infection-fighting antioxidants that ward off heart and eye disease. One carrot daily will cut strokes in women by 68 percent if combined with other responsible eating habits (Alternatives, 2014).

KALE — According to Alison Lewis, kale is considered "the new beef," "the queen of greens," and "a nutritional powerhouse" (2012). Kale is a low calorie, high fiber, zero fat vegetable—one cup has 36 calories, 5 grams of fiber and no fat, and aids digestion and elimination of waste (Lewis, 2012). Nutrient content includes folate, magnesium, and iron (more than beef per calorie), which is needed for the formation of hemoglobin and enzymes, transporting oxygen to various parts of the body, cell growth, and proper liver function (Lewis, 2012). Kale is high in vitamin K, which protects against several cancers, and is good for the bones, blood clotting, and helps those with Alzheimer's disease (Lewis, 2012).

Antioxidants include carotenoids and flavonoids which help fight against various cancers. One cup of kale is filled with 10 percent of the daily required omega-3 fatty acids, which help in the battle against arthritis, asthma, other autoimmune disorders, and also lowers cholesterol (Lewis, 2012). Its vitamin

A level helps vision and the skin, and helps prevent lung and mouth cancers. Its vitamin C helps metabolism, hydration, and the immune system. Kale has more calcium than milk to prevent bone loss and osteoporosis while maintaining a healthy metabolism (Lewis, 2012). Vitamin C is also helpful to maintain cartilage and joint flexibility. Kale is excellent for detoxing the body due to its fiber and sulfur content, which also aid in keeping the liver healthy (Lewis, 2012).

PARSLEY — Eating parsley can reduce the dangers of such cancers as skin, prostate, alimentary canal, and breast cancer because it is high in the flavonoid apigenin, which is also a powerful anti-inflammatory and antioxidant (Rogers, n.d.). The essential oil in parsley has been scientifically documented to suppress over-stimulated immune responses, such as those found in allergies, auto-immune disorders, and chronic inflammatory disorders (Rogers, n.d.). The explosive oil, eugenol, present in parsley helps reduce arthritic swelling and pain, and its folate supports heart health by lowering the amounts of homocysteine (Rogers, n.d.).

Parsley has protective properties against diabetes, atherosclerosis, colon cancer, and asthma, and as "a great generator" of folic acid, it aids in the reduction of homocysteine, a naturally occurring amino acid that can damage blood vessels when the levels are too high (which leads to strokes and heart attacks) (Rogers, n.d.). It has also been recommended as an herbal treatment for urinary tract infections. Apigenin and myristicin contained in parsley increase the productivity of the liver enzyme that detoxes the body, and its antioxidants aid in neutralizing carcinogens, might lower plaque in the arteries, and lowers blood clotting and blood pressure (Rogers, n.d.).

SPINACH — One cup of raw spinach contains 0.86 grams of protein, 7 calories, 0.7 grams of fiber, and is a powerful source of antioxidants that help defuse carcinogens and lower blood pressure (Lewin, 2014). Aside from Popeye cartoons, the high iron content in spinach has always been known to restore energy, boost vitality, and improve blood quality. "Iron plays a central role in the function of red blood cells which help in transporting oxygen around the body, in energy production and DNA synthesis" (Lewin, 2014). Spinach is also a great source of vitamins K, A, C, and folic acidas well as an equally good source of manganese, magnesium, iron, and vitamin B-2.

TOMATOES — I saved tomatoes for last because they are a fruit that is routinely treated as a vegetable. One writer referred to them as "a versatile fruit parading around in a vegetable suit" (Elliot, 1998-2014). One medium tomato contains 1.08 grams of protein, 22 calories, and 1.5 grams of fiber, contributes to a heart-healthy diet, helps protect the body from a variety of cancers, and doesn't cost a fortune, making it a flexible part of a plant-based diet. Tomatoes are high in vitamin K (18 percent of the daily requirement in each cup), which helps bone health and keeps blood vessels elastic.

Since vitamin K is stored in the body's fatty tissue, it helps to secure the calcium in the bones (Elliot, 1998-2014). As a good way to add potassium citrate (11.4 percent of the daily requirement per cup) to the diet, tomatoes help reduce blood pressure with diet instead of ingesting supplements or prescription medications (Elliot, 1998-2014). Tomatoes provide a real punch when it comes to fighting high cholesterol because they are full of lycopene, which helps lower bad LDL cholesterol while raising good HDL cholesterol.

It doesn't end there. The multi-functional tomato helps eye diseases such as cataracts and macular degeneration, and the high levels of vitamins A, E, C, along with copper, zeaxanthin, lutein, and lycopene make tomatoes a solid choice for helping the eyes stay healthy and protecting them from damage from light (Elliot, 1998-2014). There is also a belief that the lycopene alone, "or lycopene in conjunction with other phytochemicals," may aid in the "fight against pancreatic and prostate cancer as well as a number of other ailments" including lower rates of skin, pancreatic, stomach, bladder, prostate, and cervical cancer (Elliot, 1998-2014).

This list is just a sampling of what's out there in the fruit and vegetable groups to promote wellness. It might take a little discipline blended with a willingness to make the change, but you won't regret the results—a healthy body living a life of wellness.

Chapter 8

Medical Myths

The number of medical myths is so high that whole books could be, and likely have been, written on the subject. Unfortunately, there is no agreement on which is true and which isn't because no one wants to believe his/her doctor would lead patients down rabbit trails. Most of us want to believe our doctors have our best interests, ensuring our good health as their foremost concerns. For purposes of this chapter, I am highlighting some of the more prevalent myths circulating around office or hospital water coolers and, for clarity's sake, I've started with people who are often considered healthy and moved directly on to insurance companies. Don't lose heart as you read through this list.

Even healthy people can face a health crisis

The title of this section was actually a statement made by a surgeon who was talking about the wife of a Tennessee Congressman. It seems that Mrs. Congressman had been admitted to the hospital for an emergency appendectomy. Of course the statement isn't true because she wasn't the victim of an accident or a violent act and may have had surgery she really didn't need.

For several generations, medical experts held that the appendix had no purpose, but now researchers believe they've discovered the real function of the organ whereby its removal affects the immune system. Researchers at Duke University in North Carolina now know that the appendix acts as a "safe house for good bacteria" (MBD, 2013). For example, after a patient recovers from severe cholera or dysentery, which often rids the gut of essential digestive bacteria, the body sends out good bacteria that have been reserved in the appendix to restart the digestive system (MBD, 2013) (Williams, 2014).

A truly healthy person does not face such a health crisis, but even those who appear to be pictures of fitness can and often do. I have witnessed many fit, athletic individuals with various types of digestive tract ailments and worse. Former world class Olympic skater Scott Hamilton and champion bike racer Lance Armstrong have been known for incredible fitness, but even they weren't healthy enough to escape the wrath of cancer (Hering, 2005-2012). There is a difference between fit and healthy, and often those who are the most fit are actually the least healthy. Remember, wellness doesn't just mean an absence of sickness. You can appear to be fit and healthy, but you are still not well.

Illness and Health Insurance

Now let's talk about health insurance and those unpleasant, newly outrageous deductibles. When I enrolled in my employer's new insurance system, I learned that before I received any benefit from my costly insurance, I would have to meet a $3,000 deductible annually. That means my insurance carrier would pay nothing for medical care, lab analyses, tests, hospital stays, or a visit to a specialist until I met my annual deductible. The insurance company representative said the reason for this spike in costs was the high number of people who were sick last year, leading to overutilization of insurance payments.

This is absolute proof that the irresponsible lifestyles of many punish the financial health of those who are responsible about their health. How is this concept fair? It's not, but it's the new reality as the government-medical-pharmaceutical-insurance complex grows into a monster that punishes the positives and rewards the negatives. Keep this in mind as you continue to read. It may save your life and the lives of friends and loved ones in the future.

The average lifespan is 78.7 years

This number misleads people into believing they will automatically live longer, or it literally scares the stuffing out of them that they won't. In truth, it's nothing more than a medication-facilitated lifespan. That "lifespan" leads to gradual deterioration of the body via "side effects" that require additional medications to ease the original side effects created by the first medication. In other words, without medication, a re-computed lifespan regresses to the mid-50s for most Americans. This shows no significant improvement since the 1800s when the average life span was approximately 40 to 50 years of age.

Compared to other developed nations, the United States spends more per person on health care—$8,745 per capita according to an Organization for Economic Co-operation and Development (OECD) report—but our health outcomes are some of the worst (Allen, A., 2014). Further, the United States has the lowest life expectancy after age 60 and the highest infant mortality rate among almost two dozen industrialized nations (Allen, A., 2014).

I have observed many deaths among family, friends, and patients throughout my career, but have yet to know of one death due to "natural causes." According to my studies and research, death due to natural causes means that all systems shut down at the same time at the approximate age of 120 to 130 years, without the presence of pre-morbid conditions and without the presence of any life-sustaining drugs.

We have made great strides in the sciences of surgery and emergency care, but it seems we are hundreds of years behind in preventing, curing, or reversing chronic medical issues. Either our healthcare system is seriously ignorant or it is driven purely by power and profit. Considering that the average age of personnel in my department was the early 40s, it's a disgrace they suffered from so many health problems. While working at a local hospital, I closely monitored the physical therapy department's dietary habits for at least two meals—breakfast and lunch. I could easily identify the ailments from which they suffered and the ones that would impact their lives down the road.

I strongly believe in freedom of choice, but not when it directly impacts the workload and responsibilities of other workers, ultimately decreases productivity within the company, and increases insurance premiums for an entire department, company, community, or nation. It's almost as if the government is in the business of health and lifespan redistribution, deciding who will live and who will die.

Anyone over age fifty must have a colonoscopy every year

This is true if the individual follows the FDA and USDA's guidelines and consumes the Standard American Diet, SAD. However, if it ain't broke don't try to fix it. If your diet includes 95% raw fruits and vegetables and you don't experience any gastro esophageal reflux, constipation, have no history of hemorrhoids, have 2-3 soft serve bowel movements daily, and do not experience any sleep apnea, chances are that your colon is very healthy.

According to Johns Hopkins Colon Cancer Center, proper nutrition and diet are the most important ways to prevent colon cancer and to help those fighting to cure it (Nutrition, 2014). Evidence is rapidly growing that eating a healthy diet of raw fruits and vegetables provides vitamins, minerals, and antioxidants that protect the body (Nutrition, 2014). It's time to clean out the refrigerator and pantry and load up on those healthy foods.

Breast cancer patients live an average of 5-10 years longer due to early detection

When dealing with breast cancer or any other form of cancer, the media hype and the medical community seems to mainly focus on detection and treatment. There is never a mention of prevention because it is not a money maker. Study after study has proven that cancer is a lifestyle disease. It is brought on by the continued consumption of animal products and processed foods, which create an increase in estrogen levels and acidic blood—a suitable environment for the nourishment and the growth of cancer cells.

Individuals who have adopted a plantarian lifestyle following the diagnosis of different forms of cancer have been very successful in eradicating the formation of cancer cells in their bodies. Do cancer patients really live longer now? Yes and no. In most individuals, early detection makes it appear that they live longer. The disadvantage of early detection is that they live and worry longer and continue to suffer by taking on many dangerous treatments early on that may be totally unnecessary.

Medicate to "manage" high blood pressure, high cholesterol, and Type II diabetes

This is an obvious scare tactic used by the drug companies. Eighty percent of Americans take at least one medication every day, and the goal of the drug companies is to have everyone medicated daily in the near future. They are already bribing physicians to medicate irresponsible behaviors such as gambling by labeling it a disease (Wazana, 2000). Unless a situation is imminently life-threatening, medicating is bad advice. Medication treats symptoms, but only delays the inevitable. Eventually, patients experience adverse health effects while on medication but they are rarely cured.

In the United States, prescription drugs are the fourth leading cause of death, and Child Health Safety stated that "in any given month, 48% of US consumers ingested a prescription drug, and 11% ingested five or more prescription drugs" (USA's, 2012). Americans suffer from approximately 45-50 million adverse and/or side effects from prescription drugs, and "2.5 million to 4 million are serious, disabling or fatal" (USA's, 2012). With all those expensive and miracle drugs on the market, you'd think one of those drugs would be safe and make a difference—as in cure someone of some illness or disease—but they are few and far between.

Millions are currently being medicated for high cholesterol ostensibly due to an inherited disorder. Increased cholesterol production is the body's response to oxidative stress and free radicals created by poor eating and excessive exercise. Cholesterol proves vital to hormone production, and also serves as the body's defense mechanism to repair damage caused by free radicals. Medicating to reduce cholesterol is analogous to medicating to reduce white blood cells in the presence of infection—highly ignorant and completely irresponsible.

The underlying causes of infections and diseases must be found, not covered up with a pharmaceutical bandage that does more harm than good—a bandage that often works in opposition to the body's natural ability to heal itself given the right diet. Medications/ pharmaceuticals make the drug companies rich and their stockholders happy, but few, if any, will cure a condition or illness, or spare your body from the side effects from those medications. To obtain a cure, you must, as Hippocrates said. Let the right food be your medicine."

Lose weight to control high blood pressure, high blood sugar, and triglycerides

This baseless and ignorant advice has given rise to a variety of erroneous and unsafe diets, diuretics, fitness programs, supplements, and weight loss surgeries. Losing weight reduces those conditions temporarily, but relying on exercise and reduced-calorie diets as a means of losing weight can be dangerous, and the results do not last. Normalization of body chemistry, blood pressure, blood sugar, and triglycerides begins on the inside, not on the outside. It also requires adoption of a diet free of animal products and processed foods. A modified diet comprised mostly of raw fruits and vegetables directly addresses the cure for those conditions.

You must take the flu shot annually to prevent the flu

According to a report in *USA Today*, kids are the ones who the media, government, and pharmaceutical and medical industries say should get the flu vaccines (More, 2008). The article insists that this could help protect people over age 65 because that age group accounts for most of the 36,000 flu-related and flu-caused deaths every winter. The truth is the flu vaccine just doesn't protect seniors nearly as well it does young children—75 percent among children and only about 30 percent among seniors (More, 2008). Keep in mind that those vaccines are full of harmful additives, so protection comes with little or no regard for the "first do no harm" rule (Adams, 2012).

Research scientist Wilton Alston stated that "over five times as many people will die because they happen to be in the hospital and are unlucky enough to experience a preventable error, than will die from getting the flu, if the vaccine itself doesn't put them in the hospital" (2009). He also stated, " . . . [a]t best, it appears that one is opting to inject a foreign substance with likely only 25-45% effectiveness while hoping that no side-effects occur" (Alston, 2009). Considering how ineffectual those flu vaccines really are, especially as we age, and considering the harmful chemicals added to those vaccines, perhaps there are safer ways to stay healthy and well.

Drink eight to ten glasses of water daily for proper hydration

Raw fruits and vegetables consist of 70 to 80 percent water, which is harmonious with the body's water content and need for fluids. They adequately meet the body's water demands in a slower, more controlled fashion than chugging cold water. Raw foods stay in the body longer, so they better facilitate full absorption of the dense nutrients they contain, leading to better hydration. Taking in water through raw fruits and vegetables means never feeling thirsty. Most importantly, water-born enzymes flush the cells of dead, toxic, acidic metabolic waste and help keep body chemistry slightly alkaline. It is important to eat enzyme-dense foods, as they fuel the body's detoxification and elimination cycle. People remove garbage from their homes so the collection area doesn't become a foul-smelling cesspool and health hazard. The body is no different. It must be cleansed.

There are no scientific studies that support the assertion that drinking water reduces headaches or migraines, improves blood pressure, or affects skin tone. Water consumption of the recommended eight to ten glasses daily cannot perform the cell waste detoxification and elimination functions. Ingested water quickly shortens the residence time of any nutrients present in the body, dilutes stomach acids, and hampers digestion. Lastly, large volumes of water do not curb hunger. The body recognizes the empty calorie condition of the water, which signals the brain to initiate hunger pangs.

The Natural Resources Defense Council studied 103 brands of bottled water (over 1,000 bottles) and discovered that approximately one-third contained synthetic organic chemicals and bacteria - one sample even contained arsenic levels above the state health limits (Bottled, 2008). The quality of bottled water does not surpass that of tap water. In fact, in many cases, it is tap water (Bottled, 2008). Most tap and bottled water in the United States is tainted with fluoride, which is used in rat poison and is actually harmful to the development of teeth. Enamel fluorosis is the demineralization of dental enamels—the outermost layer of the teeth—and is caused by excessive ingestion of fluoride via drinking water during the years of tooth calcification (Lalumandier & Ayers, 2008).

Still, many people refuse to stop drinking tons of water. If that's the case, it's best to sip it throughout the day to increase the absorption rate. Keep the water at room temperature or warmer, but not cold. Cold water causes the body to waste energy in equalizing the water temperature to the core body temperature before its absorption. As a note of interest, it is believed that less than 10 percent of the water we drink is absorbed in the colon, and the rest is excreted by the kidneys. Drinking water may be beneficial in flushing out the kidneys and quenching your thirst but it doesn't hydrate the body. Raw fruits and vegetables do.

Back problems/other health issues are caused by poor body mechanics or unsafe work environments

While some workplace injuries do occur, most serious back injuries are not caused by lifting or handling heavy objects, and they are not caused by inherited degenerative disc and joint disease. Most result from a gradual deterioration process that precedes the actual trauma with precedents indicated by a single life-threatening malady or a combination of several. It is my observation, and that of a local and highly respected spine surgeon, that 98 percent of all serious lower back injuries, such as slipped or herniated discs, result from poor dietary health habits and an abusive lifestyle. In other words, the same lifestyle that leads to chronic dietary disorders will also result in degenerative joint diseases.

That doesn't mean workers should be careless on the job, nor does it mean they shouldn't pay attention to and employ safe workplace ergonomics. However, without a proper diet that ensures wellness, no amount of ergonomic training and practice will help if the workers are living irresponsible lifestyles and/or are making irresponsible lifestyle choices.

Life Lesson—Jason & Crew

Jason was the Corporate Safety Officer at the hospital where I was working in 2003. He wrote to me to thank me for teaching my back safety classes, my ergonomic assessments, and the nutritional suggestions I made. He wrote, "This has contributed to a healthier and more productive workforce. Your enthusiasm is contagious and employees have really bought into the lifestyle decision making. I challenge you to keep up the good work and continue to make a difference in the lives of [our] employees." Well, that letter made my day. It also helped me realize that those attending my classes were paying more than lip service when they thanked me at the end of each class. The messenger was clearly getting his message out and the recipients were taking that message to heart. So are many employers, both large and small.

In order to reduce employer and taxpayer liability, employee lifestyle and dietary habits are being closely scrutinized, since both will ultimately affect workers, co-workers, and a company's overall productivity. Further, efforts to reduce healthcare costs must take into consideration the impact of lost productivity on corporate economics—either through absenteeism or "presenteeism" (going to work while sick). A recent study by Optums revealed that losses from net productivity were anywhere from $158 to $1,601 per year for each worker with health risks or chronic health conditions (Improving, 2014). Those workers who were part of wellness programs increased their productivity and saved employers $353 annually on average (Improving, 2014). The Optum study also revealed that employees who had high-risk health issues missed work 77 percent more often than low-risk co-workers, and high-risk employees were 140 percent more likely to come to work not feeling well, making them less productive (Improving, 2014). Annual net productivity losses were $326 for each smoker, $230 for each worker with high blood pressure, and $203 for each overweight or obese employee (Improving, 2014).

Perhaps this is why employees' lifestyles are under scrutiny outside business hours. Like insurance companies who question clients about their smoking habits, weight, and other issues, some employers now screen new job applicants along with regular workers for adverse lifestyle habits and poor health. A small number of U.S. employers are taking punitive action against what they see as unhealthy behaviors. Employees might lose their jobs if they smoke or make bad food choices.

For instance, one clinic is screening potential employees for nicotine and refusing to hire those with traces found in their systems. Another health-related company plans to charge $5 per paycheck if an employee is found to use tobacco or to have high blood pressure and/or abnormal levels of cholesterol. One firm fines employees not only if they smoke, but if their spouses smoke. Though some express concern that such monitoring trends will get out of hand, most experts believe that as healthcare costs rise, employers will continue to enact penalties for unhealthy behavior.

Having been a part of a large physical therapy department of approximately 25 to 30 employees at my hometown hospital, I realized the importance of maintaining a healthy, functioning body. During my seven-year employment at the hospital, I conducted my own independent study of lifestyle habits and their direct impact on the productivity of the entire physical therapy department. On average, every employee without exception suffered at least four to five sick days per year in addition to poor productivity while at work. The reasons for the call-ins, going home sick, and lack of productivity were diet-related illnesses, which can be broken into distinct categories, though all eventually lead to and are connected to the circulatory system.

The first are what most people consider run-of-the-mill sicknesses such as nausea (unrelated to pregnancy), diarrhea, stomach viruses, common colds, the flu, sinusitis, headaches or migraines, and fevers or infections of unknown origin. The next category directly involved the circulatory system and included, but was not limited to, fainting spells, high blood pressure, dizziness, blood clots, swelling (edema), and gout.

Category three involved musculoskeletal problems such as back pain (especially low back pain), chronic joint pain, arthritis, foot pain, and tennis elbow. Add to all those conditions chronic fatigue syndrome, low blood sugar, irritability, and finally, the number two killer in America—cancer. The American workforce is not doing well with regard to health and wellness; and many of those workers might be ticking time bombs that will be set off by a major health crisis. Absent healthy lifestyle choices, it is flat-out inevitable. It's time to make healthy lifestyle choices because many of us don't even know if we are one of those physical time bombs.

No sleep/grave yard shifts and obesity, heart disease, and cancer

Let's face the facts. The night shift is not for everyone, especially those who use unhealthy methods to remain awake and alert. Staying awake during the wee hours of the night often leads to eating junk foods, drinking coffee and/or carbonated beverages loaded with caffeine, but it doesn't have to be that way. Obesity and heart disease result from poor eating, not sleep deprivation. My own observations reveal that grave-yard-shift employees suffer from excessive smoking and/or ingestion of substances that contain lots of chemicals, but little or no nutrition. This behavior is what makes them sick and increases their need for sleep. I advise you to eat the proper foods and decide whether shift work of this nature is right for you. If it's not, seek other employment opportunities before you further damage your body and your health, or endanger the lives of others, much the way those air traffic controllers endangered many lives including their own.

Enforce drug-free schools and workplaces

The "Drug-Free" regulation ignores a crucial element of drug abuse: anti-depressants, energy drinks, and foods that may lead to behavioral disorders. The side effects of illicit drugs are minimal compared to the negative side effects of legal mood-altering products. Antidepressants and marijuana allegedly make people happy, but both lead to degenerative cell damage. I do not condone taking mind-altering drugs, foods, or drinks of any kind. However, based on years of comparative study and observation of employee work performance, I have come to the conclusion that the productivity and musculoskeletal injury prevention of employees who smoke a couple of marijuana cigarettes every evening far exceeds the productivity and safety rate of those on prescribed anti-depressants or those who are suffering the consequences of bad lifestyles, especially poor food choices. I am not suggesting that you rush out and purchase marijuana. That drug may have some sound medicinal uses, but it also increases the cravings for bad carbohydrates and has its own mood-elevation and sound judgment issues that are not positive.

Cigarette addiction is tied to genes

Scientists have been honing in on finding a smoking gene that indicates the likelihood of getting hooked on nicotine for the past decade. Dr. Christopher Amos, a professor of epidemiology at the M.D. Anderson Cancer Center in Houston and author of one of the studies, states, "This is kind of a double whammy gene; it also makes you more likely to be dependent on smoking and less likely to quit smoking" (Desmon, 2008). The study, he said, also revealed that approximately 50 percent of Caucasians of European backgrounds have the genetic variation, but similar genetic studies have not been done on other ethnic groups (Desmon, 2008).

Not only do I strongly disagree with assumptions made based upon the above findings, but I am deeply concerned that this study, and others like it, may give smokers more ammunition to excuse their costly habit. In my opinion, and through studies of smokers and their lifestyle habits, I believe that, although there may be a genetic predisposition for certain destructive behaviors in all of us, it is ultimately a personal choice to carry through with those behaviors.

As stated before, I have had the opportunity to work with many patients suffering from cancers of all sorts, heart attacks, and strokes. The majority of them were former smokers for decades. It's ironic that those individuals struggled for years to stop smoking to no avail, yet they mysteriously discovered the willpower to kick the habit as soon as they experienced a serious health crisis. Although it may be too late to reverse the damage, they suddenly displayed the hidden strength they always possessed. I have also discovered that fear—and only fear—of further complications and death is the force behind the rational decision to stop smoking, not the obvious warnings or repeated pleas of loved ones.

Life Lesson—Joyce Stopped Smoking

Joyce attended one of my back safety classes in December, 2002, and wrote me a letter that had me celebrating her experience. She was extremely impressed when I explained to the class how harmful smoking is to the discs of the spine and other parts of the body, but lamented that she had tried to quit several times and failed. I was saddened that she kept seeing her attempts to stop smoking as failures when, in fact, they were valiant attempts to end a horrid habit. Well, she finally did it and stated why she made such a great decision. She wrote, "You reminded us of the most important things in our lives and how we are accountable for the choices we make. I am so glad I attended your class. It has saved my life and given me many more productive years in the future with my family."

Joyce stated that she has lots of energy and was able to exercise because she felt so much better. "Even my grandchildren can't keep up with me when we exercise. I am also more productive at work, which makes me feel better about myself." I saw Joyce from time to time and always praised her for making such a positive lifestyle choice. She reached the point of adopting the nutritional side of my teachings because she wanted to feel even better than she already did.

Of course, there are small percentages of individuals who will never give up the costly habit of smoking no matter what the consequences. Employers, however, are taking that bull by the horns. For example, on January 16, 2010, Chattanooga's Memorial Hospital took the initiative to deny employment to smokers. This policy was introduced based on the belief that smoking causes devastating health disorders such as heart disease and various types of deadly, costly cancers.

Still, my health industry experience teaches me that smoking alone does not lead to all the purported health disorders. A close observation of most smokers' eating habits can explain all of the diseases that afflict them. Few smokers say, "I've got to eat my fruits and vegetables because they're good for me." The poor eating habits that accompany smoking add to their physical devastation and leave no room for the body to recoup in any shape, way, or form.

Race may be an important factor in American infant mortality

In 2011, the Centers for Disease Control (CDC) reported that approximately 24,000 infants died in the United States, which takes a horrible toll on the well-being and health of families who suffer such a devastating loss (Infant, 2014). When a baby dies before his/her first birthday, it is referred to as infant mortality and is determined by an estimate of the number of infant deaths for every 1,000 live births (Infant, 2014). Analysts often use this rate to measure national health and well-being, and such measurements include all notable differences in infant mortality by age, ethnicity, and race (Infant, 2014). For example, the same report indicated that "the mortality rate for non-Hispanic black infants is more than twice that of non-Hispanic white infants" (Infant, 2014).

Dr. Michael Lu, an obstetrician-gynecologist and professor at the University of California at Los Angeles, studied the correlation between black infant mortality and poverty, poor nutrition, inadequate prenatal care, teen pregnancy, heredity, high blood pressure, stress, obesity, low birth weights, and prematurity (Empty, 2011). While it is true that certain races may suffer from different diseases and disorders due to their particular genetic predispositions, it is not inevitable.

As a poor young immigrant of sixteen coming to America alone from Iran in 1979, I had four important virtues instilled in me by my parents: take good care of my health, fulfill academic responsibilities, work hard, and act with compassion toward others, especially elders. Those virtues are not determined by race or sex. In my opinion, people should not conform to race labels. With the exception of people who fall victim to abuse and crime, most Americans should embrace the freedom to educate themselves and their children about responsible lifestyle choices.

Pray for good health

I believe in the power of prayer, but giving thanks for over-cooked food and saturated fat while asking God to bless your food for the nourishment of your body will not change the lack of nutritional quality. It will also not eliminate/alleviate the consequences of poor health or obesity from eating this "food." It's no different than getting behind the wheel of a car while intoxicated and praying to God for your safety. Your prayers would be more beneficial if they invoked divine intervention for the dietary know-how to set you free from the usual American diet fare.

Zoroaster, a Persian philosopher who is believed to have lived in the sixth century B.C., was likely the first ancient thinker to express the firm belief in the freedom of people to choose good over evil, right over wrong. He believed that life is a journey of choices whereby human beings choose how they will live and are totally responsible for that choice and the consequences of that choice. If you happen to believe in creationism, please realize that God loaded apples, and other natural foods like apples, with over 10,000 different nutrients. A simple prayer of thanks before eating them is sufficient because apples are already blessed since the nutrients are already there.

If you knowingly choose to ingest substances irresponsibly, my recommendation is for this prayer: "Dear Lord, please forgive my irresponsible actions in ingesting harmful substances on a regular basis, which will hold my family and my society emotionally and financially responsible for their horrible side effects and consequences." That should do it, but at that point the ball is in your court to stop your irresponsible actions and the ingestion of harmful substances. God may be longsuffering, but there is a limit.

A firm message to the men of God

Fat and unhealthy preachers, often called "men of God," should address the demon of unhealthy food choices and addictions in their own lives before demonizing others' lifestyle choices, i.e., alcohol and drugs. Regardless of whether you are thin or fat, you may be masking dangerous food addictions if you are currently taking any medications for lifestyle-generated diseases such as diabetes, most cancers, abnormal blood pressure, arthritis, or high cholesterol, to name just a few. Hold yourselves accountable to your teachings and let your flock make sure you stick to those accountabilities. It is not a laughing matter and should never be excused. Your followers, parents, and children look up to you. Don't let them down.

Chapter 9

Do You Trust Your Doctor?

The Hippocratic Oath has changed since it was first penned in the late 5th Century, B.C. The original version contained a phrase that is not in the modern version, "With regard to healing the sick, I will devise and order for them the best diet, according to my judgment and means; and I will take care that they suffer no hurt or damage" (Hippocratic, 2014). Those are great words that reveal a doctor is to "first do no harm," and that diet was extremely important to the man who is often referred to as "The Father of Medicine" (Hippocratic, 2014).

The most modern version states, in part, "I will apply, for the benefit of the sick, all measures which are required, avoiding those twin traps of overtreatment and therapeutic nihilism" (Hippocratic, 2010). It goes on to state, "I will remember that there is art to medicine as well as science, and that warmth, sympathy, and understanding may outweigh the surgeon's knife or the chemist's drug" (Hippocratic, 2010). Somehow the phrase "first, do no harm" doesn't appear in the most modern version of the oath, though my guess is it's largely implied.

However, implication is not good enough, especially since things have changed besides technology and the creation of mega institutions of alleged healing. That something can be found in the answer to a simple question: *Do you really trust your doctor?* Some folks do, while others don't. Those that don't have either done their homework and understand the medical profession or they have an inner voice that tells them when trusting is out of the question. Unfortunately, those that do trust their doctors form a far larger group than those who don't, notwithstanding my belief that there are excellent reasons not to do so.

For example, most of us have had to wait long after our scheduled appointment time to see the doctor. Waiting rooms are filled to capacity and we wonder why the wait is so long. There are several reasons why there's standing room only. It could be tardiness on the part of the doctor or an emergency that had to be handled. The first is not acceptable, the second is understandable. The usual reason given by those at the front desk is that the doctor gives each patient the time needed and will do the same for each of us, but that isn't always the truth. The truth is overbooking.

Medicine is big business and no-shows are quite common in the industry. Overbooking compensates for the no-shows by leveling the economic playing field for the doctor, but not for those left twiddling their thumbs or reading dated magazines in the waiting room or even exam rooms. I've witnessed this first hand and have spoken with patients who waited so long to see their doctors that their blood pressure wasn't even close to its normal rate. The more medicine in general and the American medical system become just another big business, the less people trust their doctors and the medical advice they're given.

One of the main reasons why some patients experience discomfort around their doctors is the "I am greater than you" syndrome, which infects the relationship. Like kings on thrones, the patient becomes the subject in a fiefdom ruled by medical elitists who want to examine your most vulnerable body parts, give you injections, and hand out or prescribe pills despite your protests to do none of what you've been almost ordered to do (Day, 2014). This leads to a greater breakdown of the doctor-patient relationship. If that trust, even false trust, is present in the relationship, it is not surprising that problems arise and a passel of truths are swept under the office or exam-room rug. But if there is little or no trust, the exam and subsequent treatments are a waste of time and money. The phrase "honest and competent doctor" is rapidly becoming as much an oxymoron as the words "honest politician" or "honest lawyer." And there are good reasons why.

According to a 2000 article in the *Journal of the American Medical Association* (JAMA) by Dr. Barbara Starfield, there were 225,000 deaths of Americans each year due to medical treatments including 12,000 deaths annually from needless surgery, 7,000 deaths annually resulting from medication errors made in hospitals, 20,000 deaths annually resulting from other hospital errors, 80,000 deaths annually from infections in hospitals, and 106,000 deaths each year from negative reactions to drugs (Starfield, 2000). You do the math. That's a quarter of a million to half a million Americans that die at the hands of the American medical system that's supposed to be healing them.

Well, what if the doctors and medical care was scarce? May be it wouldn't be as bad as you think. There have been fascinating incidents of doctors going on strike followed by decreases in the death rates. An article in the March 2012 edition of the HuffPost, UK, cited a study published in the scholarly journal, *Social Science and Medicine* (2012). Team members from Emory University and Georgetown University in the U.S. and McMaster University in Canada studied five doctor strikes that took place globally from 1976 to 2003 (Persaud & Bruggen, 2012). Doctors stopped working for at least nine days and up to 17 weeks, but the mortality rate stayed the same or was reduced during the time of those strikes, and no increases in death rates were reported (Persaud & Bruggen, 2012).

For example, the 1976 Los Angeles Count, California, strike involved excessively high medical malpractice premiums, which led to five weeks of half the county's doctors decreasing their practices and only handling emergencies. That put a big dent in elective and non-emergency surgeries, which is when a significant number of deaths occur. But when the strike was over and those surgeries started up again, the rate of deaths increased (Persaud & Bruggen, 2012).

When most workers go on strike, it's a total strike with complete worker unity, not a 50-50 split. The medical profession is different because doctors keep treating at least emergencies. A case in point: during a dispute between the Israel Medical Association and the Israeli government, 8,000 of the 11,000 doctors in Jerusalem went on strike and stopped treating patients in hospitals; but many doctors did set up "aid stations where they treated emergency cases for a fee" (Persaud & Bruggen, 2012). The mortality rate did not increase. Instead, it decreased by six deaths, and then increased by seven deaths after the strike was over.

During the 2000 strike in Jerusalem over government wages, all elective admissions and surgeries were cancelled, but emergency rooms, dialysis units, and cancer departments continued to function. Funerals decreased from 153 in May, 1999, to 93 during the 30-day strike period one year later (Persaud & Bruggen, 2012). Two theories on the decrease in death rates have emerged. The first is the realization by doctors that medicine and medical care do not have as great an impact on "mortality" as the doctors once believed. The other theory is that the striking doctors could get rid of "the shackles of its employer's restrictive practices . . . and could [practice] medicine freely, as it would really like to" (Persaud & Bruggen, 2012).

Dr. Peter Rost contends that the majority of doctors today are businessmen before they are doctors, which means medicine is now an industry that needs money to operate (Riner, 2014). What stirs the mistrust pot even more are those highly publicized incidents of fraud, drug pushing and abuse, serious malpractice, and murder committed by physicians whereby the consuming public ceases to trust all doctors, even those who have not been involved in such high crimes and misdemeanors (Riner, 2014). Add in the effects of advertising by doctors, capitation agreements between doctors and HMOs, skewed research that benefits drug companies, and lawyers advertising lawsuits on behalf of patients injured by the newest miracle drug or medical procedure, and it's no wonder the public had little or no trust in doctors or the government-medical-pharmaceutical-insurance complex that has developed over the last several decades (Riner, 2014).

What is most disturbing about that dynamic is the relationship between doctors and the pharmaceutical industry. A study, titled "National Survey of Physician-Industry Relationships," published in *The New England Journal of Medicine* and reprinted in the April 28, 2007 edition of the *Washington Post* revealed startling statistics on how dangerous that relationship has become. For example, 94 percent of doctors admit to having a relationship of one type or another with the drug industry, 80 percent of doctors frequently take free food and drug samples from drug representatives, 28 percent of doctors received compensation for consulting work, giving lectures, or getting their patients involved in clinical trials of drugs and approximately one third of doctors received reimbursement from drug companies for participation in continuing education classes or attending meetings (Campbell, *et al*, 2007).

The study also indicated a steep rise in the number of visits made by drug representatives to doctors' offices—from an average of fewer than five visits each month in 2000 to three times that average for cardiologists, more than twice that amount for internists, and nearly double that number for pediatricians (Campbell, *et al*, 2007). The only number that remained the same or lower was for surgeons.

It should also be noted that what used to be the trade of men has now become the "profession" of very attractive women. The pharmaceutical industry has chosen to sex-up the sales end of its business, which creates a possible conflict of interest for many doctors who choose specific drug therapies for their patients. Are they really looking out for the patient's best interest, or are they satisfying the bottom line for the drug companies while spending a little time with an attractive women and adding another free vacation for their obedience to the pharmaceutical company?

Here's the truth. A physician's abundant lifestyle strictly depends on your addiction to indigestible substances. Just as an auto mechanic profits from your car breaking down and would never teach you how to fix your own vehicle, the few physicians who are aware of true disease prevention will never enlighten you regarding alternatives to pharmaceutical concoctions if it will put their livelihood (and all those extra drug-company benefits) in jeopardy. Even JAMA admits that doctors are the third leading cause of death in the United States and pharmaceuticals are the fourth leading cause (Campbell, *et al*, 2007). This makes the physicians complicit with drug companies since they are the ones prescribing the drugs.

If medicine has become a high-cost industry in the United States, it's partly because physicians can no longer diagnose health conditions, diseases, or disorders without ordering a series of expensive tests conducted by other healthcare workers. The results of those tests are then sent to the physicians who prescribe drugs if the results warrant it, but the doctors are too busy to study the effects of the drugs they prescribe. Relying on information provided by drug representatives or directly from pharmaceutical companies, they will prescribe certain medications to treat a particular diagnosis. I've seen doctors become offended if a patient refuses the prescribed medication. After all, the doctor is already on his elitist throne and has no intention of letting an uncooperative patient knock him off that throne. He won't let the patient's refusal interfere with the next free vacation meeting sponsored by the drug company.

What most patients don't know is that many physicians lead very destructive lifestyles. In fact, when I look at the destructive lifestyle and job performance of a particular physician and compare it with the lifestyle and the job performance of my auto mechanic, I can't help but muster more respect and trust for the auto mechanic than the physician—and with good reason. Drug and alcohol abuse by physicians is currently at an all-time high. Approximately one out of every 14 physicians has a substance abuse problem and this has proven to be a major risk element in negligence and malpractice lawsuits (Cicala, 2003).

Physicians are people first and, like their patients who want a magic bullet to fix health problems, they may opt to take antidepressants, painkillers, or other prescription drugs in order to cope with the pressures and demands of life (Reese, 2014). Unlike their patients, however, doctors have access to a smorgasbord of medicines via their own ability to prescribe them, professional contacts, and closeness and access to hospitals and clinics (Reese, 2014). Since they know the routine so well, they are adept at hiding their addictions and will often compensate by putting in extra hours of work until evidence of their drug abuse/addiction can no longer be denied (Reese, 2014).

More obvious is alcohol addiction among physicians, especially surgeons. According to an article published by the American Medical Association, 15 percent of surgeons have an alcohol abuse problem. The study revealed that female surgeons had twice the rate (25.6 percent) of alcohol abuse compared to 13.9% for male surgeons (Krupa, 2012). The study noted that the higher rate for women was likely due to increased pressure to balance their professional lives with their personal lives, but surgeons who felt burned out or suffered from depression had a higher incidence of alcohol problems compared to surgeons who put in long hours of work (Krupa, 2012).

Finally, it is a widely-held belief that doctors detest alternative medicine options, even though they are supposed to be trained to know about the human body, how to keep us well, and how to keep themselves well. The truth is that any inspection of the medicine shelves of American drugstores would prove that alternative medicine is now an almost $50 billion industry. There is no doubt that the well-being and health of patients is the last rung of the government-medical-pharmaceutical-insurance complex ladder. The truth is that one must "follow the money." And doctors are no exception. Physicians in general are supposed to be trained to know about our bodies and how to keep us well. They should also be trained well enough to know how to take care of their own bodies. Not only do they not make us well, they tend to keep us hooked on useless and dangerous medications, and they eventually become victimized by the same diseases.

The human body wears out, begins to fall apart, or just doesn't work as well as it should. Doctors are supposed to know how to fix those problems just the way an auto mechanic knows how to fix cars. It is ironic that if your car repair person doesn't fix your car properly, he doesn't get paid. But if your doctor doesn't fix you properly, he still gets paid unless you can prove negligence or malpractice in a court of law. That says the system is upside down and proves that auto mechanics are smarter and know more about cars than physicians know about your body and/or their own bodies.

In an era when most adults don't trust politicians or snake-oil salesmen any more than they did a century ago, physicians must now make a greater effort to earn the trust of their patients. They must be vigilant regarding the profession and their colleagues, and must not allow incentives and kick-backs to influence their attitudes, behaviors, and the care they provide their patients. They must study all aspects of medicine, including alternative options and those that are still considered controversial. Equally important, they must work overtime to earn the public's respect and stop the continued transformation of a once respected profession into a government-pharmaceutical-insurance-controlled business. If anything, they must get back to the practicing of real medicine and "first do no harm" to their patients. When this happens, they can and will leave the rest of the intruders into the medical profession in the dust and start saving lives.

Chapter 10

An American Love Affair with Medications

While illegal drug use has increased in spite of the alleged War on Drugs, prescription drug use has risen exponentially over the past decade or so. In 2008, consumer and government spending for prescription drugs in the U.S. was $234.1 billion, more than twice what was spent in 1999 (Gu, *et al,* 2010). New drugs are consistently and continuously introduced into the market as the next miracle cure for, i.e., ingrown toenails. Along with this, additional uses are found for old drugs, even though the original approval of those drugs had nothing to do with those new, suddenly discovered uses.

We've already discussed the government-pharmaceutical-insurance-medical complex and the ways it harms patients of all ages. However, do we fully understand what drugs are being taken and by whom, especially since the use has increased so dramatically? According to a 2010 report from the Centers for Disease Control, the percentage of Americans who took at least one prescribed drug went from 44 percent in 1999 to 48 percent by 2007-2008, the use of two or more drugs went from 25 percent to 31 percent, and the use of five or more drugs went from 6 percent to 11 percent (Gu, *et al,* 2010).

During that same decade, one of every five children and 90 percent of older Americans stated they used at least one prescribed drug during the past 30 days, but individuals who did not have a regular healthcare facility/doctor, health insurance, or some type of drug benefit filled fewer prescriptions compared to those who did have such benefits (Gu, *et al,* 2010). Common drugs prescribed for children were asthma medications. Over the past 30 days, less over the past

30 days less than 10 percent of children under 12 made use of two or more prescribed drugs, and only 1% used five or more (Gu, *et al,* 2010).

Teenagers were a different story. The most common drugs were central nervous system stimulants (CNS) such as Ritalin and/or Dexedrine (Gu, *et al,* 2010). Middle-aged folks were having an antidepressant party while older Americans were working to lower their cholesterol with prescribed drugs. Seventy-six percent of Americans who were 60 and older used two or more prescription drugs, while 37 percent used five or more (Gu, *et al,* 2010).

Statistics from the CDC indicated that during office visits with a doctor, 2.6 billion drugs were order or provided with 75.1 percent centered around drug therapy for pain (analgesics), cholesterol/triglycerides (anti-hyperlipidemia drugs), and antidepressants (2014). Regarding hospital outpatient department visits, the number of drugs ordered for patients or provided to them was 285.1 million and 74.4 percent of those visits involved drug therapy (2014).

Drugs prescribed the most were analgesics (pain killers), antidiabetic drugs, and anti-hyperlipidemia agents to lower triglycerides and/or cholesterol (CDC, 2014). Emergency Room visits saw 271.4 million drugs ordered or provided, with 79.3 percent of those visits involved with drug therapy that included pain killers, anti-emetics or anti-vertigo drugs (to prevent vomiting or dizziness), and minerals and electrolytes (to prevent or stop dehydration) (CDC, 2014).

According to a 2014 presentation given at the *Managed Markets Summit* by Peter Wickersham, senior vice president for Integrated Care at Prime Therapeutics LLC (Prime), "the United States doesn't have a singular prescription drug problem, we have a series of challenges related to safety, efficacy and cost . . . [o]pinions may vary on the causes, severity and solutions of America's drug problems" (Prime, 2014).

Even the White House has gotten into the act, noting that, although there's been a definite reduction in the use of some illegal drugs like cocaine, data compiled for the National Survey on Drug Use and Health (NSDUH) reveals that almost one-third of individuals 12 years old and older who were first-time drug users in 2009 started with non-medical prescription drug use (Prescription, n.d.). Teens, in particular, believed that abuse of prescription drugs was safer than using illegal drugs because they were prescribed by a doctor or other healthcare professional (Prescription, n.d.). However, those drugs were not prescribed for the teens who were taking them.

There is no doubt, now, that Americans are using more prescription drugs than they did just ten years ago. Ironically, those drugs cost twice as much as they did per a study by the National Center for Health Statistics (OnlineOnly, 2015). In fact, older Americans consume the most prescription medicines, with 40 percent of seniors using "five or more prescription drugs in a one-month period" based on the number of diseases or illnesses that afflict this group (OnlineOnly, 2015).

The National Center for Health Statistics study also looked at prescription medicine usage by demographic subgroups and held that women were more inclined to use prescription drugs than were men. When researchers looked at race and ethnicity, whites use the highest number of prescription medications, while Mexican-Americans use the least amount (OnlineOnly, 2015).

Regarding the types of prescription drugs Americans used, researchers discovered that, as noted above, children were locked into use of asthma medicines, teenagers were the recipients of prescriptions for CNS stimulants, antidepressants were still the drugs of choice for the middle-aged folks, older Americans were racing for prescriptions drugs to lower cholesterol, and the drug of choice for children who were under six years old was penicillin (OnlineOnly, 2015).

The Breakthrough Care Center noted that 15 of every 1000 patients who are on medications will experience an adverse drug event each month, and approximately one third of those events could have been prevented (Breakthrough, 2014). Further, "[f]or every prescription dispensed, 25% will result in an adverse drug event in a patient within 4 weeks" (Breakthrough, 2014). Such adverse reactions and issues revolving around problems with medications has led to 4.3 million visits to doctors' offices, emergency rooms, and even hospitalizations at a cost of almost $180 billion in treatment (Breakthrough, 2014). The odds increase among those taking over six "chronic medications" or those who have complicated medication schedules, which increases the likelihood of more medical problems (Breakthrough, 2014).

David of GypsyNester.com believes America is becoming a nation of anxious hypochondriacs who, when they watch the nightly news of their choice, find out how sick they really are via drug commercials—high blood pressure, depression, asthma, erectile dysfunction, loss of hair, clotting blood, COPD, aging brain syndrome, arthritis, chronic pain, fibromyalgia, dry eyes, leaky bladder, and ugly feet (Huffington Post, 2013). The advertisements are killers, but the side effects leave most of us running away from all those pharmaceuticals, not rushing to the doctor for prescriptions.

We can thank the FDA for relaxing the rules on full disclosure of all those nasty side effects in 1997. Now, Big Pharma only has to tell you about side effects considered "serious" or "common." They don't tell you what the drug is for, they just remind you that you need it and suggest you ask your doctor about it—a way to never mention *all* the side effects they cause (Huffington Post, 2013). After a while, most Americans don't even care about the side effects; they just want the magic bullets, even if they don't work.

This makes us "the most medicated people on the planet." "Around 130 million folks take a prescription drug every month . . . [and more] than 125,000 Americans die annually from prescription drug reactions and mistakes each year," making it the fourth leading killer in the United States (Huffington Post, 2013). As Dr. Marcia Angell, former editor of the *New England Journal of Medicine,* stated "We are taking way too many drugs for dubious or exaggerated ailments. What the drug companies are doing now is promoting drugs for long-term use to essentially healthy people" (Huffington Post, 2013).

Into that environment comes even more prescription drug abuse when drugs aren't needed by most individuals at all. We are so dependent on pharmaceuticals, especially prescription drugs, that we're becoming a nation of drug addicts. In fact, the classic drug abuser "could easily be your next-door neighbor, the teen who babysits your kids or the grandmother you chat with at the grocery store . . . because drug abusers could be abusing the medication they bought at the local pharmacy" (Montgomery, 2014).

According to the National Institute on Drug Abuse (NIDA), the most commonly abused prescription drugs fall into three categories—opioids (pain killers such as codeine, oxycodone, and hydrocodone), depressants that affect the central nervous system (Klonopin, Valium, and Xanax), and stimulants that enhance brain activity (Dexedrine and Ritalin) (Montgomery, 2014). The reason for the exponential rise in prescription medications and their abuse has been blamed on easy availability via the Internet, but it's also laid at the feet of the baby boomers that now comprise a large senior population for whom painkillers and pain relievers are prescribed and abused (Montgomery, 2014).

The National Institute on Drug Abuse states that the elderly are approximately three times more apt to use prescription drugs and don't always follow dosage instructions. They are also given higher doses of some medications and for longer periods of time (Montgomery, 2014). The elderly are followed by healthcare workers who have easy access to all kinds of medications and prescription pads (Montgomery, 2014).

In 2010, *U.S. News and World Report* revealed that 61 percent of adults are taking at least one prescription drug to treat a chronic health issue, up 15 percent since 2001, and 25 percent of seniors are consuming a minimum of five medications per day (Kotz, 2010). Poor dietary choices have led to rises in diabetes, heart disease, obesity, and arthritis, and revised guidelines put out by Big Pharma have led to a proliferation of drugs to deal with high blood sugar, high cholesterol, and hypertension (Kotz, 2010).

Meanwhile, experts are concerned that many individuals are taking unnecessary drugs that may have unknown long-term consequences - even though clinical trials say that they are safe (Kotz, 2010). Such was the case with Vioxx, an arthritis prescription that caused "between 88,000 and 139,000 heart attacks during the five years it was prescribed" (Kotz, 2010). Experts have strongly condemned the FDA for its poor drug safety monitoring practices once they're on the market because ongoing studies are conducted by the drug companies who set the tone for any additional research—and it's always in their favor (Kotz, 2010).

Conversely, we must not forget our own responsibility for protecting our first line of defense, regardless of the FDA's shortfalls. Arthritis is the result of poor or inefficient nutrients circulating in the blood, which means individuals who took those drugs were already at high risk for heart attacks, strokes, diabetes, cancer, and other life-threatening or chronic diseases. It is also likely that those individuals were also on a series of prescription or over-the-counter drugs to mask other chronic ailments. While Vioxx may have played a role in those heart attacks, it was not the main, underlying reason they occurred. Adverse side effects from drugs manifest themselves in several ways—drug to drug, drug to food, and drug to specific disease. Placing full blame on Vioxx as the only cause of the heart attacks experienced by Vioxx users negated the main reason people took the drug—the quick fix.

OTCs (Over-the-Counter) Drugs

OTCs are totally accessible, somewhat affordable, and provide consumers with the power to choose the remedy they believe will do the trick. However, OTC use is not as benign as people think it is. According to the Consumer Healthcare Products Association, approximately 70 percent of parents have used OTC medicines at night to treat the onset of a medical problem, and 81 percent of adults turn to OTCs as the first option for treating minor illnesses. This means that 60 million people get some type of relief of symptoms from those illnesses (CHPA, 2015).

The nitty gritty on OTCs is that Americans "make 26 trips a year to purchase OTC products," but only see the doctor about three times per year. With about 54,000 pharmacies in the U.S., there are over 750,000 retail stores that sell OTCs (CHPA, 2015). The healthcare industry saves $102 billion per year, $77 billion in clinical costs (no doctor visits or diagnostic tests), and $25 billion in drug costs (CHPA, 2015). However, like many prescription drugs, OTCs cure nothing, they only treat the symptoms - and many can do more harm than good.

The National Institute on Drug Abuse holds that "prescription and over-the-counter drugs are, after marijuana (and alcohol), the most commonly abused substances by Americans 14 and older" (NIH, 2014). The most widespread abused OTC drugs are cough and cold remedies that contain dextromethorphan and, as with any drug, when OTCs are abused, they can cause addiction and adverse health problems including overdoses. This is especially true when certain OTCs are taken with alcohol or other drugs (NIH, 2014).

For example, if dextromethorphan is consumed in very high doses, it affects the same cell receptors that are affected by PCP or ketamine and the abuser can suffer the same type of out-of-body experiences (NIH, 2014). Dextromethorphan can also cause weakened motor ability, numbness, and nausea and/or vomiting, an increased heart rate and blood pressure, and possible hypoxic brain damage. The latter is caused by intense respiratory depression and lack of oxygen to the brain, which can happen when dextromethorphan is taken with decongestants that are usually found in the medication (NIH, 2010). All drugs, including OTC products, can lead to addiction, a risk that's increased when they are abused.

When you switch to a plantarian diet, your body operates at optimum wellness, which makes it unnecessary to take most of the prescribed or OTC drugs. Does it mean you'll never get sick? Not a chance! However, it does mean that all your body systems are operating at full speed and have the ability to ward off illnesses that affect most people at one time or another.

Chapter 11

Let Food Be Your Medicine

Again, the words of Hippocrates ring true—"Let food be thy medicine and medicine be thy food." This was how people healed themselves. Their food kept them healthy and contained medicinal qualities, and if they did get sick, the same food contained the nutrients needed to heal them. We're not as smart today because we think that science is ahead of the curve.

If you're not afflicted by acidic body chemistry, high blood pressure, high blood sugar, or high triglycerides yet, you need to adjust your lifestyle - especially if processed foods dominate your diet. A diet loaded with processed foods creates chemical dependence on those products and the chemicals within them, which leads to the deterioration of health and wellness.

The good news is that gaining more energy, rebuilding the immune system, and regenerating organs is possible, as is reversing the health effects from acidic body chemistry, high blood fat, high blood pressure, high blood sugar, and all the diseases caused by those four conditions. Embrace a diet comprised of at least 95 percent raw fruits and vegetables, then balance out the rest with processed food choices, preferably cooked vegetables, which are the least damaging of all processed foods. I call this the 95/5 split, with 95 percent of your intake leading to wellness.

That split lets you take control of your diet *and* destiny by minimizing the intake of processed simple carbohydrates and animal protein in the diet—a vital component of truly healthy living. There is sound reasoning and science behind recommending a diet of predominantly raw fruits and vegetables. The enzyme and nutrient composition of raw fruits and vegetables are ideally compatible with your body's chemistry. It will also help your body fight disease and begin to reverse a host of diseases and conditions you were never meant to endure.

Life Lesson—Jean K.

Jean followed my nutrition suggestions and stated that she reduced her blood sugar and didn't require insulin as often. Her blood pressure was steadily coming down which led to her doctor cutting the dosage of one of her blood pressure medications in half. Her energy level was up and she lost six pounds. All of this took place one month after our discussion.

How Things Work

There is a science to the way things are laid out in this world, including how people and animals should eat. For example, the Earth is composed of 60-70 percent water. Raw meat is also 60-70 percent water and is a major source of enzymes (USDA, 2011). Wild animals eat their food raw. Carnivores' teeth are long, sharp, jagged, curved, and blade-shaped, while their claws are sharp for tearing. They possess speed and power to hunt and kill their prey. With regard to body chemistry, carnivore saliva contains no digestive enzymes, and the small intestines are three to six times its body length. The colon is simple, short, and smooth. What goes in doesn't hang around for long, but is eliminated in a timely manner.

Animals that live, hunt, and eat in the wild do not become obese, and they don't die from diabetes and other diet-related diseases. They also don't cook their foods. I've never seen a lion or tiger, wolf, pack of dogs, or a pod of stray cats cooking their meats over a roaring campfire and neither have you. Cooking meat depletes it of its enzymes (Dehydrated, 2014). Human beings, on the other hand, have much to learn about eating and wellness.

Like the planet on which we reside, the human body is 60-70 percent water, but we cook our foods. Human teeth are broad and flattened, like all grazing animals, and we have fingers and hands for picking and gathering food—no speed, power, and claws to hunt prey. Human saliva *does* contain enzymes that digest carbohydrates. The intestines of human beings are 10 to 11 times the length of the intestines of herbivores, animals that are anatomically and physiologically accustomed to eating plant material. The human colon is long and complex, much like the colons of all grazing animals. So, if you thought humans were carnivores, you are wrong. We are omnivores, which is defined as an animal or person that eats food of both plant and animal origin. This is based on all relevant anatomical traits, and before processed foods and junk foods became staples of the American diet, the blend worked. It doesn't anymore. While we are smarter than animals, or operate based on intellect far more than instinct, most of us die from numerous diet-related diseases because we are no longer eating real food.

Aside from large and small bodies of water (salty or fresh), the high percentage of water present on the surface of the Earth—and in both animals, humans, and fruits and vegetables—suggests that humans and animals were designed to eat raw foods as a primary source of nutrition. Somewhere along the way, man discovered fire and learned how to cook animal flesh and vegetables. While it probably depleted nutrients and enzymes from their diets, it was at least real food. However, once man started to eat processed foods and excessively processed carbohydrates, mankind started to regress, rather than progress, and a host of illnesses began attacking the human body.

Food For Thought

Animals, unlike their supposedly smarter human counterparts, obviously don't cook the essential enzymes and nutrients out of their food. Lions eat animal protein without getting fat or contracting diet-related diseases because their protein intake is *raw*—straight from a kill. They don't eat kibble packaged in fancy packages replete with advertising claims. Wild animals don't have to put up with equally annoying and deceptive advertising campaigns created by processed food manufacturers, bargain product sales, fast food franchises, vending machines, or government manipulations. That explains why news reporters never feature wild animals eating at a local fast-food restaurant or suffering from diet-related diseases, and only a cartoon tiger claims to eat sugar-coated cereal. There is no Type II diabetes epidemic in the wild animal kingdom. There is no Type I diabetes in young animals because the expectant mothers eat nutritiously.

For instance, bears gain fat prior to hibernating. During hibernation, they lose weight because the enzyme lipase breaks down fat and burns calories, eliminating waste. Gorillas don't get fat because they eat an unprocessed vegetarian diet that provides a sufficient amount of protein for their enormous muscles. The common denominator for animals in the wild is that their diets consist of raw carbohydrates or proteins, not the cooked and processed foods Americans love. There has, however, been a rash of diabetes cases among domestic pets because most eat processed pet foods.

Clinical science has determined that cooked and processed food groups overwhelm the digestive and immune system over time. Meat needs an acidic enzyme for metabolism. Complex carbohydrates need an alkaline enzyme. Acid neutralizes alkalinity, which slows digestion and results in overstimulation of the endocrine gland system. The body expends enormous amounts of energy-secreting enzymes to digest cooked and processed food groups. That's why people want to sleep after eating. Their energy has been used up digesting and confronting the stress afflicted at the cellular level by processed food.

According to nutrition expert Lisa Guy, "When we feel overly tired after eating, it can be related to eating processed foods that contain high levels of sugar and refined carbohydrates" (2014). Consuming those types of foods causes an increase in blood sugar only to be followed by a drop that causes lower energy levels (Guy, 2014). When excessive secretion of insulin occurs, the body is trying to balance its levels of blood sugar. This causes tryptophan to move into the brain where it is turned into serotonin and melatonin, neurotransmitters that create calm and regulated sleep (Guy, 2014).

Let's Talk Motivation

Many people lack purposeful motivation, a condition that enablers work hard to maintain. This is closely related, in most cases, with low self-esteem, which can cripple one's physical and emotional health, and rob a person of potential if it's not resolved. In order to rebuild self-esteem and embrace wellness, one must first retrain and change his/her "mindset." Putting the ideas that follow into practice and making them part of your life is essential to altering unhealthy/stale lifestyles, which leads to higher self-esteem. You must engage in dream-building, develop the ability to focus, create positive imaging, develop a support system, have a role model, and have a reward system.

Dream-building is an integral and required part of how one goes about achieving success at any task. This applies to a range of things, including repairing self-esteem. Dreamers need a mental image of what they want to achieve. Once they have that image clearly defined, they must identify and separate, in proper sequence, the component parts of the dream. This starts with the foundation elements. One must repeat this same process, moving through the dream in a vertical direction until reaching the peak of action and imagery.

The process of identifying the component parts of a dream require scheduling time to focus, shutting out all distractions, and devoting perception to the task at hand. Removing distractions and negativity helps us maintains focus. The degree of success attained is in direct proportion to one's ability to disengage from the environment while staying positive. When you achieve a relatively steady state of positive thoughts, you break the ties that bind you to unhealthy living and life becomes a more enjoyable experience with fewer struggles.

The components of the formula for success may seem egocentric, but small doses of egocentricity are essential to one's health, self-esteem, and overall sense of wellbeing. This is a small price to pay because a lot of adults devote their lives and existence in service to everyone else but themselves. Being other-centered is, for many, an appropriate way to live because they have the tools—mental, emotional, and spiritual—to live that way. However, dream-building is a small self-indulgence and really not so egocentric when considered in the overall context of life. It is an investment in one's identity. As Hillel the Elder stated, "If I am not for myself, who will be for me? If I am only for myself, what am I? And if not now, when?" Hillel understood balance between the self and others.

The next step is dream reality. Family and peer support are important to stay motivated and positively egocentric. Seek support from those who encourage, inspire, and motivate. Find a friend dealing with the same or comparable challenge, who is also a positive role model. Choose someone who has been successful in rebuilding self-esteem, in wellness, and in lifestyle change. This serves as a progress benchmark. Egocentricity is good and not an occasion for embarrassment. Everyone is special and has something unique to offer this world that nobody else possesses.

The final motivational technique comes from a reward system that is not steeped in food. Start with a small, non-food reward—something that feels like a treat—such as a facial, massage, a new outfit, or a weekend vacation. Remember, a reward system does not prevent or protect against setbacks. They happen to everyone, but that's no reason to give up the whole journey. Setbacks do not define progress! Aim for the greatest reward: a healthy body that looks good on the inside and on the outside while achieving smaller rewards in the process.

This works for everybody

During my career in health care, I've worked with all kinds of patients seeking relief from chronic diseases. I've met people who are wealthy or poor, educated or illiterate, well-connected or isolated, highly athletic or physically unfit, spiritually redeemed or spiritually wicked. The common denominator that places those people next door to each other in hospital rooms at any age seems to be poor diet, which I call The Great Equalizer. The food choices made today shape future potential and opportunities, no matter who you are or where you are on the economic, educational, fitness, or spiritual ladder of life. Programming the mind for success doesn't happen without work, because the human mind does not work involuntarily. A person must engage and make conscious, repeatable efforts to act and think in a healthy manner. Repeating healthy actions and thoughts on a daily basis turns them into habits and guarantees success. The behavior modifications in the section that follows will help keep you on track.

Behavior Modifications

Step One

Energy, health, and quality of life dramatically improve by reducing the percentage of processed foods containing saturated fats, simple carbohydrates, trans-fats, and animal protein to no more than five percent of daily intake. Some fat is necessary for digestion and vitamin absorption, but the source should be the mono-unsaturated type that comes from complex carbohydrates found in raw foods.

For wellness, people should minimize eating anything that is cooked or that comes in a bottle, box, can, or cellophane wrapper. When you adopt this lifestyle, the body receives the protein, carbohydrates, and other essential nutrients it requires. Initially, on a diet comprised of healthy foods, an overweight body will lose three to five pounds a week in water weight due to a decreased consumption of processed salt and sugar and improved heart and kidney function. Water loss can represent between 20 and 30 percent of total excess body weight. Subsequent weight loss will result in the reduction of actual body fat over a longer period.

Step Two

Stopping or dramatically reducing alcohol consumption makes total sense. Alcohol offers no nutritional value; it only contributes empty and damaging calories. It is absorbed rapidly in the bloodstream as sugar, causing wild swings that stress the body to produce insulin, thereby weakening the immune system. Alcohol also destroys liver tissue and shortens one's lifespan either through serious illnesses, liver failure, or intoxication-related accidents.

Step Three

Excess salt consumption damages health and leads to water displacement from the blood supply into the surrounding tissues. This results in the classic case of swollen ankles and other extremities, also called edema. It ultimately leads to low blood volume, increased blood pressure, and dehydration, which reduces the ability to be mobile without discomfort or pain.

Step Four

Stimulants damage health. Caffeine and ephedrine found in popular drinks or diet pills jump-start the central nervous system and cause excretion of adrenalin and other hormones. The secretion of adrenalin and hormones stresses the body by increasing the heart rate, blood pressure, and blood sugar. Both take their toll on the adrenal glands down the road, as well as affect vessels and arteries, resulting in coronary heart disease. Stimulants are also linked to heart arrhythmias.

Step Five

Sugar and all sugar substitutes cause numerous health issues. Consumption of sugar is synonymous with empty calories, dangerous water retention, and weight gain. It causes dangerous levels of sugar to rise in the bloodstream. This cascades to the endocrine section of the pancreas (the islets of Langerhans), which must produce insulin to metabolize the sugar. As the sugar level recedes from the action of insulin, hunger and weakness set in and the cycle starts all over again. Sugar also impairs heart and kidney functions, resulting in fluid retention. Since sugar substitutes originate in a laboratory and not in nature, my advice is not to use those products. A limited amount of real sugar doesn't hurt every so often, but *every so often* means just that. One should not use it on a weekly basis, and you should never use sugar substitutes.

Step Six

Smoking stresses the body by increasing heart rate and blood pressure, constricting arteries and vessels, and increasing the likelihood of blood clots. It also increases homocysteine levels in the blood, which leads to acidic conditions. With every drag on a cigarette, you are inhaling toxins like acetone, ammonia, hydrogen carbon monoxide, cyanide, formaldehyde, radioactive polonium sulfide, and vinyl chloride. This habit victimizes families and societies and comes with a high price. It isn't easy to quit smoking, but I never recommend one take drugs to do it.

There's an old saying, "Plan what you do, and do what you plan, and if you fail to plan, you will plan to fail." This book provides the plan, which consists of a determined willpower and a healthy diet. The plan is difficult at first, but recovering from cancer or taking the first step after a stroke is much more difficult. If it were easy, everyone would be healthy. Falling off the wagon with a cigarette will happen. It should not lead to regular smoking and falling back into old eating habits that are detrimental to your health and wellness. The important thing is to get back up and keep eating raw fruits and veggies to diminish the addiction. It takes commitment, chemistry, and time to train the body to stop the nicotine cravings.

I suggest everyone read these steps on a daily basis, or as often as needed, to achieve a dream reality that makes you glow with health and happiness. You won't be sorry, and your dreams will become reality while you're awake, not just when you're sleeping. Now that's a huge bonus to add to all the other bonuses you'll accrue in the long run.

Chapter 12

Becoming Obese

With an understanding of how digestive enzymes and antioxidants work to enhance health, the next step to overcome dependence on processed foods is to identify and confront the origins of obesity. The truth is: obesity has never killed anyone! *The underlying health problems that lead to obesity kill people.*

Genetics do not provide a total solution. I agree with most medical experts that obesity is a behavioral disorder, and while the incidence of true genetic obesity exists, it is rare in comparison to environmental influences. Genetics determine our predispositions. Individual choices convert predisposition into reality. Bear in mind that genetic changes take place over time, whereby diabetes, coronary heart disease, and cancer have replaced infectious diseases as the major causes of death.

It is equally true that the environment plays a part in obesity. If your family members are all obese, and if they subscribe to the "big is beautiful" mantra, then you have a greater chance of adopting that body style and mindset without batting an eyelash. Further, for the sake of argument, if obesity was genetic then people with that predisposition would not be determinants of their own destiny. That assumption flies in the face of the fact that the Creator endowed all with free will.

According to an August 15, 2013, study published in the *American Journal of Public Health*, obesity is linked to almost one in five deaths in the United States, which indicates that obesity's toll on American lives is three times greater than prior estimates (Laidman, 2013). Previous studies that minimize the effects of obesity on American lives have been countered by Ryan K. Masters, PhD, a Robert Wood Johnson Foundation Health and Society Scholar at Columbia University's Mailman School of Public Health in New York City (Laidman,

2013). Masters and his colleagues reported that overweight and obesity were linked to 18.2 percent of all adult deaths from 1986 through 2006 in the United States, notwithstanding a 2009 estimate published in *Demography* claiming that deaths related to obesity were only five percent of all adult deaths (Laidman, 2013). The differences are attributable to a lack of consideration by 2009 researchers of lower participation in public health surveys by the obese as well as the reliance on average rates of obesity, which "blur the substantial differences among various age groups" (Laidman, 2013).

In a study conducted by the National Cancer Institute (NCI), researchers noted that people with class III obesity, or extreme obesity, experienced a striking decrease in life expectancy when compared with people whose weight was normal (Laidman, 2013). The findings, published in the July 8, 2014, issue of *PLOS Medicine*, revealed that extreme obesity is increasing to the point that six percent of adults now have the distinction of being considered extremely obese, meaning their weight is more than 100 pounds over the recommended range for normal weight based on average height (Laidman, 2013 ; Kitahara, 2014).

The Mechanics of Overeating

The hallmarks of obesity include a diet that's dependent on processed foods, an empty immune system, and oxidized, acidic body chemistry. When those conditions take root, the obese condition increases rapidly. The pure mechanics of how one overeats originates in the endocrine glands and central nervous system. Both systems communicate with the brain's hypothalamus, signaling when hunger has not been satisfied. Leptin is the protein circulating in the body that signals the hypothalamus when fat cells are full. When ingested food lacks enzymes to support the endocrine gland system, opioids are emitted to stimulate the appetite and cause a hunger craving. Eating enzyme-diminished/acidic foods causes opioid production to peak. This condition leads to overeating, enzyme reserve depletion, chemical dependence, and acidic body chemistry. When overstimulation occurs, some 4,200 calories from processed/cooked foods are required to satisfy the hunger signal from the hypothalamus.

Life Lesson-Bernard's Story

I met Bernard, a 63-year-old Black man, in September of 2011, when he was a physical therapy patient. My experience with Bernard was somewhat different than my experiences with my other patients. He was extremely polite and intelligent, but at 425 pounds his health was rapidly declining, he was bed bound, and basic functional mobility was extremely difficult for him. Bernard was totally dependent on his loyal and caring wife; and he was very depressed due to his chronic pain, total dependency on others, and the heavy dosage of pain killers he was taking to tolerate his severe low back pain. He explained that he had been on insulin to control his Type II diabetes and high blood pressure medicine since 1975.

I immediately connected with Bernard when I realized that, notwithstanding his poor state of health, he still volunteered his time to help people who had been wrongfully terminated from their employment. I was on a similar page, fighting for people who were destroying their health due to their own ignorance or wrong health advice. I knew that physical therapy alone was not the solution for this impressive man. I talked to Bernard and his wife for two hours about ways to improve his health. He became very excited about the information I was presenting to him. He had always been told by other health professionals that he needed to lose weight, in part because his race makes him more susceptible to the chronic diseases from which he was suffering.

My message was far different from the advice he had been given all his life which got his attention. His weight was never an issue and I was not interested in addressing his weight loss. Instead, I presented a plan to improve the health of his vascular system. I guaranteed him that if he stuck with the new eating regimen, he would be able to reverse his diabetes and hypertension even though he was told his pancreas would never produce insulin again and he would need insulin injections for the rest of his life. There wasn't much I could do to fix his degenerative spine condition which was caused by years of poor lifestyle habits. However, his vascular disease could be reversed which would make his mechanical issues, especially with his spine, more tolerable; and if he chose to undergo back surgery, he would be much stronger physiologically and far more able to handle the procedure. While I told him how to perform some exercises, including safety instructions, to satisfy the physical therapy requirements, I knew that was not what he needed to achieve wellness. I left him, not knowing whether he would follow my suggestions.

Two days later I went to see him again. Bernard stated that after my talk, his wife became very excited, rushed to the grocery store, and came back with lots of fruits and vegetables. He stated that his wife cut up the produce for him and he started to eat raw fruits and vegetables for breakfast, lunch, dinner, and for snacks in between the meals. I made another physical therapy visit a few days later and found that he was very depressed. He could hardly stand on his legs because of his severe spinal degeneration, pain, and morbid obesity, and had lost all hope of ever walking again. Further, he was scheduled for an MRI of his low back, but transporting him down seven steps by EMTs would cost an additional $1,200 not covered by insurance. That meant he would never be able to leave the house to get treatment.

Based on my experiences with white Americans, I decided to challenge Bernard's "race related" diseases. I promised him that if he adhered to my dietary proposal (95% raw fruits and vegetables and 5 % cooked vegetables), he would be able to walk down the steps on his own, in six months. Bernard agreed to take the challenge with a renewed hope. In three months Bernard was able to discontinue his insulin and his blood pressure medicine. His nurse practitioner was amazed; but I wasn't surprised. I had witnessed many of my patients reach such goals as part of their journeys to wellness.

Bernard began his journey in late September, 2011; by late March of 2012, he was able to walk down his seven steps, while holding onto the rail. He was amazed and very excited about his new found freedom. I personally transported him to the hospital to weigh him on a special scale. He had lost nearly 65 pounds and went on to lose nearly 120 pounds in a year. We still maintain contact and after four years he is still free of his insulin and high blood pressure medicines. He is one of my favorite success stories.

Obesity in the Black Community

While I never focus on the race of my patients, having seen people of all backgrounds, obesity is far more common among African-Americans than any other ethnic group. The latest statistics reveal that they are 1.5 times more likely to be obese compared to white people (Desmond-Harris, 2012). Some experts claim that upbringing and culture are part of the problem while others believe that blacks were raised eating foods that were high in sodium, fat, and/or sugar (Desmond-Harris, 2012). Another problem appears to be availability of healthy foods as well as the affordability of those foods.

Dr. Tyeese Gaines has reported that over two thirds of African-Americans over 20 years old are either overweight or obese, which means their Body Mass Index (BMI) is 25 pounds or more (2010). For example, BMI charts reveal that a 5-foot 5-inches tall woman who weighs 150 pounds is overweight, and a man who is 5-feet 8-inches in height is overweight at 175 pounds (Gaines, 2010). Even this amount of extra weight creates a greater chance of developing Type II diabetes and hypertension, both of which disproportionately affect black adults and children (Gaines, 2010).

Sadly, many blacks see larger size as culturally acceptable because curvy, overweight women are considered more appealing to black men than normal- or under-weight women (Gaines, 2010). That leaves obese women in that culture struggling to lose weight while thin women strive to gain weight which is why "4 out of 5 African-American women are overweight or obese" (Gaines, 2010). In fact, according to Gaines, "Regular exercise, portion-control and healthy eating habits are not routinely ingrained into the structure of African-American families" (2010). Further, Type II diabetes and hypertension have trickled down to the children who are also overweight which only acts to continue the obesity cycle. Add to this the tradition of eating "soul food" which includes recipes that have been passed down through the generations, and you have a cultural obesity epidemic that is destroying all members of black families.

The California Food Guide indicates that African-American cooking tends to include foods like yellow and green leafy vegetables which are nutritious and high in vitamins and antioxidants. Other traditional foods include low-fat, high-protein items like fish, poultry, and beans. Unfortunately, the cooking process includes deep frying, using ham or ham hocks to season the foods, or soaking foods in gravy. This flies in the face of all heart-healthy recommendations which include reduction of the intake of sodium and fat (Cowling, 2006). As Linda L. Cowling, M.P.H., R.D. noted, "Many African-American rites revolve around food . . . [and the staples] of soul food include fried chicken, fried pork chops, cornbread, and ribs. Many of these dishes use large amounts of pork fat, butter, and salt for flavor" (2006).

Further, baiting of blacks by the fast-food industry creates a recipe for disaster that's cooking on the cultural stove. This was recently documented by Sam P.K. Collins who reported that from 2010-2012, researchers at Arizona State University studied over 6,700 fast food restaurants that were chosen from a national sample of over 400 communities with high populations of middle school and high school students (2014). Those restaurants that were "located in middle-class neighborhoods, rural communities, and majority black neighborhoods used child-directed marketing strategies more often than their counterparts in non-Hispanic and majority white neighborhoods" (Collins, 2014). This type of marketing to children only adds to the obesity problem in black and other minority families and fosters eating habits that lead to serious illnesses in both the adults and children living in those cultures.

Life Lesson—Gail Makes a Change

Gail was also an attendee at one of my back safety classes, which incorporated healthy eating with back health. She wrote to me several years after taking that class, "In the past 7 years, I have slowly gained weight and have tried numerous times to shed my extra 20 pounds! As a Type II diabetic for the past 22 years, I realize the importance of maintaining my optimal weight . . . to avoid medication and the complications of diabetes." Since November 14, 2004, Gail modified her diet using my nutrition suggestions, specifically my recommendations for breakfast foods. She incorporated more vegetables and fruits, less meat, and avoided rich, high-fat food sources. She lost seven pounds, had more energy, required less sleep, and her ankle joints were no longer stiff upon arising in the morning. "Thanks so much for getting me back on the right track! Your nutrition plan is working for me when nothing else did!"

Nothing else worked for Gail because the process was never properly explained to her so she could put it into practice. What she didn't know is what most people don't know—that oxidization from a depleted-enzyme diet causes the body chemistry to change from normal alkaline to acidic. Eating processed foods compromises the body's defenses. It eliminates antioxidant action for free radical neutralization, enlarges glands and organs, and reduces the body's ability to ward off diseases. In this stressed condition, the body responds by becoming sluggish, achy, and tired. Insulin, produced by the pancreas to metabolize sugar, stimulates the production of the enzyme lipase, which then absorbs fat in the bloodstream. Fat storage is measured by increased body weight. If the body's fat storage capacity exceeds 85 percent, new fat cells are created to accommodate the overload. Fat cell production and storage in water is a stressed, acidic body's natural defense mechanism. The body stores fat with water to help buffer acidic components to maintain an alkaline environment.

On the flip side, storing fat with water creates water retention, increased weight, and swelling. Incidentally, other causes of swelling or water retention include sugar and salt, which, when regularly consumed in processed foods, create a displacement of water in the cells and the blood. Salt and sugar move into the cells and blood and force water into the surrounding tissues. The individual then becomes dehydrated, which leads to low blood volume and eventually hypertension. This is not a condition that can easily be corrected by overconsumption of water or any other fluids and it exemplifies the definition of water weight.

The health of the body thus deteriorates, and when the body is no longer able to store fat, it enters the bloodstream as triglycerides. Insulin emitted from the pancreas is absorbed by fat in the blood, which effectively blocks the metabolism of sugar. As a result of insulin absorption by fat, sugar levels rise in the blood stream. Sugar that is not metabolized causes a variety of problems for the body, from retinal eye damage to blindness.

Life Lesson—Lula Sheds Pounds

Lula also changed her diet and wrote of the drastic improvements in her health: "I lost nearly 40 pounds, I don't have to take Lortab or sleeping pills at night, and am no longer suffering from constipation." Her insulin component went from 75 units to 5-10 units per day, her headaches stopped due to lower blood pressure, and with less swelling in her legs she could walk without joint pain and shortness of breath. Her sister was totally impressed, started following my dietary recommendations, and noticed the benefits almost immediately.

The Body Processes

In a healthy body, minor amounts of fat and cholesterol from animal protein are converted by a healthy immune system. An unstressed liver converts cholesterol into bile acid to facilitate digestion. If the liver is already over-stimulated or exhausted from eating enzyme-depleted foods, cholesterol conversion to bile acid stops. Cholesterol subsequently begins to accumulate in the blood, veins, and arteries. This condition meets the requirements for the onset of symptomatic high blood pressure, high blood sugar, and high triglycerides.

Alternatively, eating foods that are high in nutrients and complex fiber provides considerably fewer calories that can be converted into body fat. Raw foods are not only the easiest to digest, they also facilitate their own digestion because they are rich in enzyme content and other micronutrients. Five hundred calories of raw, enzyme-rich food will satisfy a hunger craving because raw food is high in enzymes, as well as insoluble and soluble fiber. The high fiber in raw food has nine times the volume found in processed food. The difference in food volume supplied by the high fiber signals the brain that the stomach is full and the required enzymes are sufficient in quantity. Eating raw food requires less energy for digestion, sparing more energy for enjoying life and being productive. As an added benefit, enzymes burn a greater number of stored fat calories to digest raw food.

Proof of this has been seen in studies on animal diets and nutrition and the emergence of raw-food diets for even domestic pets. Dr. Ian Billinghurst, a veterinarian and leading advocate of the raw-foods diet (called BARF/Bones and Raw Foods or Biologically Appropriate Foods), calls this diet "evolutionary nutrition" because wolves are the ancestors of today's dogs (McKenzie, 2010). While the appearance of dogs has changed over the centuries, there's been no change to their basic internal physiology, which means their food requirements and other needs haven't changed (McKenzie, 2010). Holistic veterinarian Dr. Richard Pitcairn notes that all processed pet foods are missing the same "nutrient" as foods processed for human ingestion—"life energy" (Pitcairn, 2005). Maybe we should listen to the vets. If we're willing to consider raw diets for our pets because it's healthier and prevents obesity and the diseases that either cause it or stem from it, why not do the same for ourselves and our loved ones?

Some folks were brave enough to give it a try. In a January 11, 2007, BBC news report, nine British volunteers, age 36-49, experimented with an ape-like diet for twelve days to decrease their blood pressure and cholesterol levels (Heald, 2007). Their temporary home was a tented enclosure right next to the ape house at Paignton Zoo, Devon, England, and the whole experiment was filmed for TV (Heald, 2007).

Jill Fullerton-Smith, who assisted in the organization of the experiment, stated that modern diets are often dominated by processed foods and saturated fats, which lead to expensive health problems (Heald, 2007). The diet regime was developed by Lynne Garton, a nutritionist and registered dietician, and King's College Hospital. The nutritionist and the hospital used research that showed the diet might work because it was comprised of foods the human body evolved to eat—in this case eleven pounds of raw fruit and vegetables daily. Volunteers were allowed to drink some water and during week two were given some cooked, oily fish reminiscent of the hunter-gatherer style of living (Heald, 2007). At the end of twelve days, the volunteers had decreased their cholesterol and blood pressure levels. On average, they noticed a ten-pound weight loss, a twenty-three percent drop in cholesterol levels, and a decrease in blood pressure from 140/83 to 122/76 (Heald, 2007).

Perhaps we can learn from that "eat like an ape" experiment, and do our bodies a big favor and join in the fun minus the tent or cage. Poor lifestyle choices that lead to obesity take the joy out of living, destroy our health, and put us at risk for many other serious health conditions. This kind of lifestyle doesn't sound like the best way to journey through life. Instead, take a journey to wellness to make life completely worthwhile.

Chapter 13

Reality Check—Exercise, Weight Loss, Obesity

Obesity, in some ways, has become an epidemic in America, even with all the hype about diets and exercise. Some say it's really a political football with many (mostly on the left) screaming that obese people are discriminated against on a regular basis. While some claim obesity is genetic, others prefer to rename it "caloric overconsumption" or "excessive energy input"—the outcome of activity or behaviors, not the cause (Shelley, 2012). However, choosing to be obese doesn't just affect the individuals who make that choice, it affects society by promoting self-discrimination more than external discrimination. It also results in the obese avoiding activities and relationships that make life worth living.

Many heavy people do not date or have sex, play sports, or even travel long distances because it's hard to fly anywhere when seats don't come in jumbo size. Just walking through a store brings on episodes of panic and use of a motorized shopping cart provided by stores like Wal-Mart or Target. Obesity interferes with creating strong ties to the community and loved ones because life is all about focusing on and managing fat.

It's embarrassing for an obese person to talk about a new love interest or the possibility of a dinner and/or movie date when restaurants and movie theaters do not have chairs or seats that can accommodate the obese person's size. There's also no way to explain that a walking tour of a new city sounds perfect, except for the walking. Forget public and private swimming pools, lakes, or ponds, because, even if obese people have the courage to wear a bathing suit, they know they will receive stares from other swimmers and sunbathers due to their weight.

I have had experiences working with many morbidly obese men and women who have health problems lurking under the folds of their skin. In some cases, it's yeast and in other cases it's bacteria. Sometimes there is a combination of the two because the folds of skin create a dark, moist area for both organisms to grow. I have also personally found crumbled food from past meals eaten in front of the television or in bed, remote controls, cell phones, and other items in these folds, and the individual doesn't even realize they are there.

Obesity is not a case of "marching to the beat of a different drummer," so if the claim is discrimination, the claim is not true. What is true is that people tend to reject those who are deliberately unhealthy, and that's how many view obese people. Being fat cuts down on almost anything except eating and, in many cases, labored breathing, and it costs the rest of society a lot of money. According to a report by the Milken Institute, decreasing the obesity rate to the 1998 level would save $60 billion in annual healthcare costs and increase productivity by $254 billion (Milken, 2008). Obesity does make people different, and it affects everyone else around them. Glorifying it with slogans like "big is beautiful" do nothing to help the obese person and only enrich companies that thrive by making clothing for oversized people.

So how do we care for our bodies so we do not become obese, and how do the obese tackle their obesity? Everyone has a theory, a magic potion or bullet, a super-terrific diet, or an exercise plan or surgery that will do the trick. Sadly, the number of myths is off the charts when it comes to exercise, weight loss, and obesity. I will deal with a handful of the most common myths, but you are free to explore further. In fact, I encourage you to do just that.

Cook healthy meals to lose weight

There is no such thing as a "healthy cooked meal," especially a "healthy cooked frozen meal," but it's true some cooked foods are worse than others. However, that's not what the diet gurus and weight loss companies want people to think because they sell cooked meals. Some cooked meals are just not as damaging as others depending on the saturated fat, sodium, and sugar content.

It is also true that cooking food using any method is going to have a negative impact upon its nutrients, and fewer nutrients are lost the less the food is cooked (Sexton, 2011). The key element involved in loss of nutrients is heat, and the amount of nutritional value foods lose during the cooking process is directly related to how long they are exposed to heat—this is especially true for vegetables, fruits, and meats (Sexton, 2011).

With Americans suffering from obesity, heart disease, and a host of other diet-related diseases, the practices of marketing, accessing, and delivering unhealthy cooked foods to the public for profit is almost a crime. Eating cooked meals on a regular basis from infancy to old age is a prescription for chronic and/or catastrophic illnesses. A cooked meal offers empty calories that tax and weaken the immune system by forcing it to deplete the body's reserved enzymes and vitamins to digest the food instead of utilizing those micro/macronutrients to boost the immune system and subsequently protect the body from disease. This process opens up the opportunity for nothing but long hospital stays over time.

You can stay healthy by counting calories, fat, points, and carbohydrates

David B. Allison, PhD, is the Director of the Nutrition Obesity Research Center at the University of Alabama, Birmingham. He recounts the story of a woman who told him how she was eating all the "right" foods such as whole grains, fat-free dairy, and fruits and vegetables, but was not losing weight. While he didn't discuss the food groups, which were nothing to write home about, he did counsel her on the difference between healthy food and energy or calorie content (Allison, 2014). It is his belief that people have lost weight on diets that were rich in foods thought to be healthy, while others lost weight on the latest fad diets that restrict calories—the high-fat-low-carb diets, low-fat diets, and even on diets of only McDonald's or only Twinkies (Allison, 2014). All of those diets are equally unhealthy, even though a few consider calorie content.

People who want to starve while losing weight should pay attention. Those who don't want to waste away into wisps of their former selves have a better option—switch to a diet of predominantly raw fruits and vegetables that doesn't require any bookkeeping talents, graph reading, or counting skills. The simple reality is that raw plant foods do not cause the body to gain excess weight because they contain the enzyme *lipase* which metabolizes fat and ***prevents its accumulation*** in the fat cells of the body. So, it's time to grab an apple and keep reading.

Eat according to your blood, body, or metabolic type

Most of the Internet research on metabolic typing, blood-type diets, and body-type diets is what we would call "old news." There is very little current literature on such diets, but the old information still touts those methods for weight loss as miracle methods. The truth is that the body's responses to poor dietary choices depend on its predisposition or certain weaknesses at the cellular level. Current thinking purports that a simple-carbohydrate diet of cooked or processed foods will fuel those predispositions and weaknesses and lead to diseases. On the other hand, the body's response to a healthy diet never varies. It's always positive and not likely to facilitate diseases at the cellular level regardless of any physiological variations or genetic predisposition.

Poor nutrition habits are considered a behavioral health issue because a person's diet affects how that person looks, feels, thinks, and acts (Ajmera, 2013). A bad or unhealthy diet leads to reduced core strength, less alertness, a slowdown in the ability to solve problems, and altered muscle response time (Ajmera, 2013). Forget the fad diets. They may work for a short time, but they do not produce permanent results unless you make them a total way of life.

You must schedule your meals and eat at the same time every day

The digestive organs respond to enzyme-depleted or enzyme-rich foods in the same way at all times. A high-fat, processed meal or snack will tax your system at 10:00 a.m. in the same way and intensity as it will at 11:00 p.m. On the other hand, consuming enzyme-rich raw fruits and vegetables all day never stresses your system and is very beneficial at any time of day.

The author of *10 Habits That Mess Up a Woman's Diet*, Elizabeth Somer, M.A., R.D., believes we should eat when we're hungry, not when a clock says we're hungry and should eat (Bouchez, 2005-2014). There's nothing wrong with some consistency with regard to mealtimes, but Somers believes that you could be forcing yourself to eat or not eat if you eat by the clock. Either way, no diet can be successful under such conditions. However, when there's a designated lunchtime at work, relax and eat the next meal when your stomach tells you it's time to eat (Bouchez, 2005-2014).

Weight gain is caused by slow metabolism

I once heard a morbidly obese registered dietician say she was fat because of her slow metabolism. Even more disturbing and irresponsible was the fact that the hospital allowed her to instruct patients in dietary guidelines. Appearing to be at least one hundred pounds over her ideal weight, she had surpassed the state of "fatness" and earned the status of morbidly obese. Likely, she subscribed to the propaganda regarding fast, medium, or slow metabolism disseminated via the media and even scientific journals - but it's just not true. In fact, many obese people have faster metabolisms than those whose weight is healthy. Still the lies continue with obese people believing that thin folks have "won the biological lottery" because they can eat anything and everything they want and not gain weight (20/20, 2006).

To understand the myth of metabolism and weight gain, 20/20 sought out Dr. Jim Levine, who researches obesity at the Mayo Clinic and studied the metabolism of thin and fat people. Levine found that heavy people actually have higher metabolisms than thin people because metabolism is actually the calories burned to keep the body going (20/20, 2006). Dr. Donald Hensrud supports this reality, holding that a slow metabolism is rare and isn't the likely cause of being overweight (Hensrud, 2014). It is his contention that rather than slow metabolism, weight gain is likely caused, in part, by eating too many calories, family history (your diet growing up), certain medications, lack of sleep, and unhealthy habits (Hensrud, 2014). Unless you have hypothyroidism or Cushing's syndrome, your metabolism is probably high if you're obese.

The real truth is that the metabolic rate increases as stress on the body increases. When the body suffers chronic stress, it attempts to achieve physiological neutrality by increasing metabolism. Chronic stress leads to depletion of stored enzymes and nutrients, and over time it will lead to a depressed immune system, thus inviting a host of diseases such as cancer, diabetes, heart disease, and obesity. Normalize your metabolic rate by lowering the physiological stress at the cellular level through proper food consumption and less strenuous exercise.

Weight gain is an inherited trait

This statement illustrates the highest form of denial. Weight gain comes from poor food choices. Each processed meal acts as a building block that causes addiction to saturated animal fat and simple carbohydrates. This leads to overconsumption of saturated animal fat, sugar, and other highly-refined simple carbohydrates, the latter being the prime factor in cases of obesity. It takes very large quantities of processed food to satisfy hunger cravings because the nutrients have been cooked out. Cells remain unsatisfied, leading to the beginning stages of clogged arteries and increased body mass in the future.

To prove my lack of bias on the issue of hereditary obesity, I found two sources that point to *underlying* hereditary issues that can lead to obesity, but that also prove my point about healthy eating. A recent study conducted by researchers at King's College in London, U.K., and Cornell University, New York, U.S., revealed that bacteria naturally found in the gut involved in obesity, diabetes, and cardiovascular disease are genetically inherited (Moss, 2014). This inherited bacterial family of microbes called Christensenellaceae and other microbes were far more similar in identical twins than non-twins in the study, which indicated a strong genetic influence in microbe composition in the gut (Moss, 2014). My first question would be, "How did those microbes get there in the first place?"

Reporting on the same study, Dr. Charlotte Warren-Gash claimed that genetic make-up does influence the type of bacteria that live in the stomach, which may play a part in weight gain (Warren-Gash, 2014). However, while the study included 416 sets of twins who were raised in the same environments, researchers were quick to pinpoint the cause of those microbes in the gut as hereditary, which may be a stretch.

Where is the information regarding the diets of those twins while they were growing up, and why is the presence of Christensenellaceae so high in some of the study subjects in the first place? Since they can't prove that obesity, per se, is hereditary, scientists found a little microbe in low amounts in obese people to claim that heredity is involved. The scientists involved in the study want us to believe that genetics, and only genetics, accounts for the presence of those microbes, but I'm not buying it. What if their presence is due to diet and/or environmental factors? Perhaps the reason for the hype is because people are champing at the bit to create new probiotics—the proverbial magic bullet—filled with the little critters to help obese people lose weight. Follow the money! You're bound to find the truth.

Stress can cause weight gain

Stress results in weight gain only when foods with low-nutrient density are ingested during stressful times. Daily chronic stress leads to the overproduction and release of hormones such as adrenaline, epinephrine, and cortisol. Those hormones are responsible for breaking down glycogen into glucose. Modern stress differs from what ancient humans experienced. Family, jobs, money, and relationships bring on stress that many deal with inappropriately. It is not the stress that causes poor health, but the body's secondary reactions to stress, such as comfort eating, that lead to detrimental health.

The truth of this has been born out by medical professionals. Some researchers believe that weight gain when under stress might be partly the result of the body's "system of hormonal checks and balances," which causes stress-related weight gain (Stoppler & Shiel, Jr., 2014). However, most people confess that when they're under stress, they find it hard to maintain a healthy diet or healthy eating habits (Stoppler & Shiel, Jr., 2014). They either eat to deal with emotional needs or fill up on fast foods because they don't have the time to make something healthy to eat (Stoppler & Shiel, Jr., 2014). Eating unhealthy is the cause of the weight gain, not the stress. The one time your body needs to eat super healthy is when you are under stress.

Obesity is contagious

A July 2007 study in *The New England Journal of Medicine*, which was noted in the July 25, 2007, edition of *The New York Times*, held that individuals whose closest friends are obese increase their own risk of obesity (Kolata, 2007). This may be true, providing those individuals are easily influenced by peer pressure, misinformed, or ignorant of the consequences. The study also indicated that the tendency to become obese when a friend became obese increased by 57 percent, but there was no effect when a neighbor gained or lost weight. The same held true when family members were involved (Kolata, 2007). Ironically, it didn't matter whether the friend lived nearby or at a considerable distance because the issue was mutual closeness in the friendship. In that case, the odds of joining the friend in the obesity trap almost tripled (Kolata, 2007).

My own experience with this type of situation occurred several years ago when I began dating a young woman whose lifestyle included eating out at least once or twice a day. Prior to meeting her, I preferred to eat out no more than once a week. Since I enjoyed her company, I started to meet her at different restaurants once or twice a day for breakfast and lunch. Although she was not obese, she suffered from multiple ailments such as the loss of her gallbladder, occasional migraines, and numerous episodes of dizziness and nausea. She was also easily irritable, all of which could have stemmed from poor dietary habits.

I realized that my own health and body were slowly deteriorating from such a destructive relationship. In ten short months, I gained nearly ten pounds and felt sure that it wouldn't take long for me to suffer from the same or similar health disorders. I was forced to end our relationship in order to protect my health, respectability, and to continue fulfilling my duties as a parent, productive employee, and wellness instructor at the teaching hospital.

There's no harm in being a close friend to an obese person or someone suffering from other lifestyle choices such as smoking. But if one's own lifestyle and health begins to spiral downward as a result of the friendship, and all possibilities to improve the situation have been exhausted, then the relationship must end. This holds true for couples with regard to body size, notwithstanding known health consequences. For example, many times I have been told by women, "My husband likes me better as a big woman." If your spouse truly loves you, he or she shouldn't expect you to have a diseased body just to provide them with temporary physical satisfaction.

Exercise more/eat less

A pediatrician in Chattanooga, Tennessee, stated at a Children's Wellness Seminar that when her son asked for some ice cream, she would have him do a few chin-ups before he was allowed to eat any. I also heard a physical therapist co-worker say, "I exercise and jog a lot because I know I eat horribly." These are the people in whom we entrust our health and lives as well as those of our loved ones. If they're not qualified to take care of themselves or their own loved ones, how can they even come close to caring for others?

Exercise is beneficial for muscle maintenance, strengthening, and flexibility. It also helps with relaxation and, to a limited degree, circulation. Exercise doesn't reduce, eliminate, or neutralize the chronic illnesses and harmful chemicals in processed foods. Regular strenuous exercise can promote or speed up the degenerative process and the onset of chronic illnesses due to increased metabolism, subsequent surge of free radicals, and physical wear and tear on the joints. In fact, "eating less and exercising more have consistently been proven to FAIL for more than 95% of the population" (Bailor, 2014). Eating less is bad advice because the body needs nutrient-dense, raw foods for cell nutrition, elimination processes, and waste detoxification to maintain a strong immune system. Nutrient-dense foods are high in soluble and insoluble fiber that fills the stomach and produces a full feeling. Starving hurts people, physiologically, mentally, and physically.

Jog your way to good health

I began getting interested in jogging as a teenager in 1977 in Iran. I also encouraged some of my friends to jog with me late at night, even with a military curfew during the Islamic revolution. I continued with occasional jogging after I came to the U.S. because jogging made me feel good and I felt like I was doing something very healthy for my body. However, in early 2000 when I was turning 40, I realized that jogging may not be what the body really needs to maintain good physical health. Throughout my career in physical therapy, I learned to protect my health by doing the exact opposite of what my patients were doing. I had the opportunity to treat many avid joggers who were in their mid-40 and 50s. Those individuals appeared to be healthy, but their continuous and severe aches and pains would land them in the hospital for low back surgeries, hip and knee replacements, and ankle reconstructions. They were subjected to the same procedures as my severely obese and unhealthy patients.

I soon realized that the human body is not designed to be jogging or running for hours at a time. It's no different than driving your car for more hours than just short everyday trips to prolong its life. It doesn't work that way. I knew many joggers who appeared to be intelligent individuals based on the academic degrees they held, but they took pain medications so they could tolerate joint pains. Some would even wear ankle, knee, or back braces while they jogged. I didn't want to deal with aches and pains in my 50s, and though I was always a fast sprinter, I also didn't want my aches and pains to diminish my ability to win100-yard dashes against people 10 to 20 years my junior. This led me to analyze jogging from the physiological stand point.

It is clear that cellular activities require oxygen, and it's logical that more strenuous activities require more oxygen. As the oxygen use increases, so does the carbon dioxide output by the lungs and the cells. The carbon dioxide output is also known as cell waste, oxidation, or free radicals. Continued exposure of the cells to free radicals is responsible for cell degeneration of all tissues, organs, and systems in the body. Further, increased cell waste, or free radicals, is directly related to increased ingestion of processed foods and strenuous exercises such as jogging. Both place a physiological demand and stress on the body.

Free radicals are partially neutralized only by the presence of antioxidants. Antioxidants are only present in raw fruits and vegetables. They are not present in capsules, pills, drinks or powders. You cannot find them at health food stores or physicians' offices. They are found only at produce stands or the supermarket produce department that occupies only 10 percent of all grocery stores, including the so-called fresh or whole food markets.

Jogging produces not only physiological stress and degeneration, but also mechanical stress to all weight-bearing joints including hips, knees, ankles, and the spine. As I compare jogging to cigarette smoking, I cannot help to realize that the free radical or oxidation accumulation may be similar. Smoking introduces the free radicals in the smoker's body, but jogging manufactures the free radicals with an added detriment—wear and tear of the weight-bearing joints at an early age.

I stopped jogging in early 2000 and I am still very active without experiencing joint pain. At age 52, I continue to be a fast sprinter—faster than people half my age. My exercise regimen consists of minimal resistive exercises and occasional bicycle rides. I don't have a need to jog long distances or build big muscles by lifting heavy weights. If I need to travel far enough from my home, I drive my car, and I move my refrigerator or other heavy objects with my two-wheeled cart. It's called being smart and using common sense. It's also called wisdom not to adopt the newest health fad because it might very well be dangerous to your health.

No pain, no gain

Staying active and stretching is great for toning and stress release. However, many fitness instructors use this dangerous philosophy as a mantra. Pain is one of the most primal response mechanisms in the body. Pain is bad, yet it is also good. Without pain sensation, a body wouldn't survive. Pain during exercise means the body is sending an alarm message to cease and desist.

When trauma occurs to the fibers in your muscles, nociceptors (pain receptors) in muscle tissues are stimulated and your brain then feels the sensation of pain (Greenfield, 2013). Further, when muscle tissues are being torn up, the calcium normally stored around your muscles accumulates inside the injured muscles (Greenfield, 2013). This accumulation can activate enzymes called "proteases" and "phospholipases" that can break down and degenerate muscle protein, causing inflammation and further pain due to the accumulation of inflammatory and pain-producing chemicals such as histamines and prostaglandins (Greenfield, 2013). Ignoring the pain by continuing the behavior or medicating are bad choices and lead to unwanted, serious complications. If a person routinely experiences pain during exercise, he or she should decrease the intensity and the frequency, or consult a qualified healthcare professional.

Sometimes diet and exercise don't work

This statement qualifies as one of the most irresponsible and supremely deceptive statements I have ever heard from a healthcare provider, who just happened to be a gastric bypass surgeon. I couldn't believe it when he said it. His demeanor reminded me of a sleazy used-car salesman. Obesity is an irresponsible behavioral disorder, and an anatomical modification by way of invasive procedures such as gastric banding, sleeve, or gastric bypass fails to alter such behavior.

Personal tragedies, such as the loss of a loved one or a divorce, may induce temporary weight loss. A gastric bypass procedure is a self-induced personal tragedy that results in short-term weight loss by creating a dangerous dysfunction. That dysfunction is the malabsorption of essential nutrients. A voluntary decision to undergo such surgery leads to a whole host of ailments, since over 80 percent of immune systems are developed in stomachs and digestive tracts that depend solely on the types of food consumed.

Many doctors, hospitals, and even the FDA promote this and similar immuno-suppressing surgical money makers. Most regrettably, such procedures have become fashionable for teenagers who see it as an easy resolution to their weight problems. According to a study by the Agency for Healthcare Research, the number of candidates for the surgery increased by fourfold between 1998 and 2002 due to a 2,000 percent jump in the number of patients between the ages of fifty-five and sixty-four (Obesity, 2007). Gastric bypass has been even more profitable for the hospitals, which generated over $1.3 billion in 2004 from the procedures, complications (27 percent of complications are difficult to diagnose due to the massive size of the patients exceeding the weight restriction for the imaging equipment), and follow-up plastic surgeries to remove the excess skin folds (Obesity, 2007).

People think of extra weight as a monkey on their backs, but this surgery produces huge gorillas. Only 10 percent of those undergoing gastric bypass sustain weight loss. Forty percent to 50 percent experience complications following the surgery, with a two percent to three percent mortality rate, in addition to temporary or irrepressible weight loss in the long run (Gastric, 2005). The procedure offers other long-term side effects including bone loss, dumping syndrome, hair loss, recurring diarrhea/vomiting, and vitamin depletion, to name just a few.

In my opinion, this procedure is more like a punishment than a treatment. If those procedures succeeded as promised, lobbyists for the restaurant and food industry would bring this practice to a screeching halt. A better alternative would be to have a limb surgically removed. That guarantees weight loss without all the serious complications or hospitalizations.

Financial incentives can motivate employees to lose weight

Paying employees to lose weight can seriously backfire and create unhealthier employees, especially when the employees are allowed to follow a diet of their choice. Such a contest, "Wellness You," was put together in March 2005 at the hospital where I worked. The contest was initiated by a group of registered dietitians and approved by the administration. Ironically, the lead registered dietitian supervising the competition was suffering from poor lifestyle choices and morbid obesity.

According to a few employees who entered the contest, the registered dieticians did not offer the contestants a sensible lifestyle to follow. They were encouraged to follow the everyday fad diets such as Atkins, Jenny Craig, and Weight Watchers. Furthermore, the contestants were not closely monitored. According to my sources, some of the contestants (including the winner) used dangerous and risky means to lose their weight and win a prize.

Life Lesson—Susan & Company

As managing partner of a local law firm, Susan was thrilled with my ergonomic assessment of the firm's staff. She was equally thrilled with my seminar on back safety, nutrition, overall health and wellness, and lifestyle changes. She wrote, "The facts and information you provided and specific physical instructions were not only eye opening and helpful, but your overall presentation was interesting and fun. I am confident that our employees will make workplace and lifestyle changes as a result of your efforts and that they will be healthier and thus more productive at work and at home." She also noted, "James, as you know, we had a lot of lawyers and staff participate in the ergonomic assessment and seminar. On behalf of each one of them, thank you for showing us how to take better care of ourselves." Again, I was the messenger who shared the truth with them. When a bunch of lawyers and their staff react positively, you know you've done something right.

This is a perfect example of how employers should deal with colleagues, associates, and all others working for the company. To improve employee health, a company must present the long-term impact and benefit of a healthy lifestyle, showing the direct effects of improved habits. To be effective, it is imperative that employers educate their employees by way of a true and unbiased wellness program that helps improve productivity not only at work, but also in other areas of life. The most important fact to realize is that weight loss does not lead to wellness. Only wellness does.

Limiting a child's time in front of TV prevents obesity

I agree whole-heartedly that spending long hours in front of the television is not the healthiest activity for a child's mind and doesn't build socialization skills. But I have never known of a single child who got fat simply by watching TV.

After my divorce, the custody and care of my children was granted to their mother. This meant I no longer had much control over their lifestyle and dietary habits. My children's physical, emotional, and academic health was deteriorating before my eyes, and the legal system's impotence was unable to protect their rights. To make matters worse for my children, the judge ruling on my divorce was suffering from his own lifestyle diseases, such as Type II diabetes. There were days he was absent from the bench due to his uncontrolled blood sugar, which I believe was the result of continued irresponsible eating habits or following his health professional's bad advice, or both. He was of no use to my case when he was present due to his irritability and obvious lack of desire to be there.

Almost two years later, I regained full custody of my children. My son had gained approximately 10 to 15 pounds of unhealthy weight due to poor eating habits at home and school. Even though he was attending one of the most prestigious elementary schools in town, the food there was just as unhealthy as that offered at the public schools. I began working to improve his health. In order to accomplish this task, I had to eliminate all outside influences such as school lunches and other junk foods.

The summer of 2003 offered the opportunity to do just that. I purchased a new computer for him with all the bells and whistles. I turned him loose in front of the computer and offered him mainly raw fruits and vegetables without a regular exercise regimen. To keep him from feeling deprived, I offered him fast food twice a week. He lost fifteen pounds during that summer. He lived with me for nearly ten years, and during those years I was able to lead him into a reasonable and nutritionally responsible lifestyle.

However, TV does present other dangers and most come from the advertisements that promote candy, fast foods, sugary cereals, and toys. The American Academy of Pediatrics has noted that "adolescents and young adults who recognized TV ads for quick-service restaurants were more likely to be overweight" (Familiarity, 2012). So while watching TV doesn't lead to weight gain, leaving children unattended in front of a television is no different than allowing a salesperson to come to your door and ask for a few moments alone with your children to promote their products. The process of brainwashing starts as soon as the child is old enough to turn on the tube. Children become familiar with different junk foods on TV, and they badger their parents until they get what they want. The moral of this story is that watching TV does not make our children fat - typical American foods and marketing do.

Now that you know the truth about obesity, diets, exercise, healthy eating, and wellness, what will you do? If you are obese or need to lose some weight, will you take the challenge and change your current eating habits before it's too late? And if you're not overweight, will you do what it takes to achieve true wellness? I cannot answer that question for you, but I will continue to provide honest information that you can use to guide you on your own journey to wellness.

Chapter 14

Coronary Heart Disease

Deposition Kinetics

Oxygen is necessary to support life, but as with all things in nature, an opposite effect can occur. Oxygen from an acidic, processed food diet has an oxidative effect on our bodies. This results in the generation of unstable radicals that are at the heart of diet-related diseases. You are about to learn all the information your physician doesn't share with you. Brace yourself. It's really very straightforward and meant to scare the processed foods, saturated fats, and bad carbohydrates out of your diet.

The process begins early on with a diet containing saturated and polyunsaturated fatty acids (PUFAs). As the years pass, calcified plaques form an unhealthy lining inside the arterial vessels like sludge in the pipes of a house, and lipid (the general name for fat of any group of organic compounds) peroxidation begins to inflame the interior surface of the artery wall. This is initiated by the presence of PUFAs that are attracted to free radicals.

When free radicals react with PUFAs, a chain reaction known as lipid peroxidation (LPO) is initiated. LPO can also be attributed to oxidized cholesterol from cooked (i.e., pasteurized) milk and other animal foods; the absence of antioxidants, such as vitamins A, C and E, and the presence of high levels of homocysteine (an amino acid in the blood that lowers blood pH); and tobacco smoke, which increases homocysteine levels in the blood. It also drains the body's resources of antioxidants, particularly vitamin C, further accelerating arteriosclerosis. Many smokers also eat poorly, which accelerates the process.

Lipid peroxidation damage to the arteries and vessels begins with the removal of orbiting valence electrons (oxidation) from atoms comprising the artery and vessel tissue. This leaves a scar that constitutes a change in electro-chemical potential at the scar site where it previously exhibited a neutral charge. Based on the difference in charge, calcium and oxidized cholesterol are electrically attracted to the site and are incorporated into the scar tissue. When calcium predominates, this process is called "hardening of the arteries," or arteriosclerosis; when when cholesterol predominates, it is called "atherosclerosis."

According to researchers, high blood cholesterol increases the risk of certain cancers by repressing an important protective protein known as TGF-beta that functions as a tumor suppressor (Link, 2007). The exact amount and content of the plaques are determined by the individual's diet, antioxidant fruit and vegetable intake, and duration of the process. Regardless of where on the arteriosclerotic/atherosclerotic continuum an individual falls, the result is the same. The tissue between the deposit and the artery surface site where the plaque has accumulated becomes deprived of its normal oxygen supply (Link, 2007).

Prevention of Cholesterol Deposition

Shifting to a plantarian diet can control the cholesterol buildup of these plaques. Liberal intake of antioxidants, including beta-carotene (the precursor of vitamins A,C, and E found in plantarian foods), halts lipid peroxidation. The body cannot manufacture these micronutrients, nor can they be supplied through health food store supplements, so they must come from the diet. Antioxidants safely interact with free radicals and terminate the chain reaction before vital molecules and cells are damaged. Additionally, selenium, a trace metal required for proper function of one of the body's antioxidant enzyme systems, is sometimes included in essential micronutrients. However, reversal of cholesterol deposition is possible.

Chelation is an acid-based chemical reaction that results in a bond between a metal ion and an organic triglyceride, or between a metal ion and cholesterol molecules by sharing electrons from the outer shells of atoms. The resulting complex of metal bound to molecule is called a "chelate." The complex contains one or more rings of atoms in which the metal ion, such as calcium, is so firmly bound it cannot escape. This allows calcium in cholesterol deposits to be combined and moved just as you would move water through a hose. This process is called "natural chelation." It is totally compatible with human body chemistry if the source is from natural raw produce.

Natural chelating acidic agents are found in abundance in an enzyme-dense diet of raw fruits and vegetables. For example, citric acid from citrus fruit is a strong chelating agent used for years to remove metallic calcium from water piper, which is likely why all those citrus cleaning solutions were dumped on the market over the past decades. Natural chelating agents from whole fruits and vegetables, along with their nutrients, safely penetrate the blood brain barrier and perform the same type of body cleansing.

Life Lesson—Thomas & Triple By-Pass Surgery

When Thomas had triple by-pass surgery, I was his physical therapist assistant and talked with him about making needed lifestyle changes, especially his diet. He was overweight, a smoker for more than 50 years, had high blood pressure, and suffered from Type II diabetes for which he took Glyburide 5mg once each day. That's when Thomas decided to stop smoking and embrace a plantarian lifestyle. He lost 40 pounds, his blood pressure was under control, and his doctor told him he no longer had diabetes. "I am still working on further improving my health and general lifestyle. I heartily recommend you and your program."

Artificial Chelation Is Not Safe Chelation

Artificial chelation is a man-made process with varying and some yet-to-be-known side effects. This chemistry often involves using weak, manufactured organic acids like ethylene-diamine-tetra-acetic acid (EDTA) to treat lead or mercury poisoning. EDTA in the presence of some natural chelating agents is also being practiced around the country as a means to eliminate artery and vessel blockage. Laboratory-produced EDTA is introduced through intravenous injection. A single treatment session lasts approximately three to four hours, and patients may receive up to thirty treatments in the first month at a cost of $50 to $100 per session (not reimbursed by the insurance companies).

This definitely generates significant revenue for practitioners of "chelation therapy." However, it's not the way nature intended to remove deposits from the human body, especially since it's not scientifically verified or validated. Clients who seek such treatments suffer from a list of associated diseases caused by artery blockage that restricts the fresh supply of oxygenated, nutrient-bearing blood to organs and vessels. However, artificial chelation without adequate and balanced nutrients could result in a dangerous drop in blood calcium levels and a rise in heavy metals and minerals such as zinc.

EDTA is a drug that may cause side effects such as kidney failure and can also lead to allergic reactions, bone marrow depression, convulsions, low blood pressure, irregular heart rhythm, respiratory arrest, and shock. A significant number of deaths in the U.S. have been associated with chelation therapy (Chelation, 2010). A number of health issues also factor into this equation. For example, true Alzheimer's disease is mimicked by simple arterio/atherosclerosis of the arteries and arterioles supplying the brain. Natural chelation through consumption of proper nutrients can prevent such an unforgiving disease.

Cholesterol deposits in people with all types of diabetes results in poor blood flow to the pancreas. This can decrease output of digestive enzymes from the exocrine part of the pancreas, causing incomplete digestion. Poor blood supply to the stomach and small intestines results in poor digestion, and poor blood supply to the colon slows the organ's movement, resulting in colon disease and an increased likelihood for colon cancer.

Decreased blood supply to the kidneys results in the inappropriate release of angiotensin, a peptide hormone that constricts blood vessels, inducing hypertension throughout the vascular tree. The joints, particularly the weight-bearing joints, including those in the low back, react with inflammation and pain. This, along with the degeneration of ligament tissue and disc disease, is responsible for the so-called "low back syndrome." Arteriosclerosis/atherosclerosis also plays a big part in the onset of arthritis throughout the body.

The effect of this process on the heart is angina (chest pain originating in the heart) and, eventually, heart failure. The effect on the limbs produces cold hands and feet and, in advanced cases, limb amputation. Impotence can be caused by decreased blood flow to the penis due to clogged arterioles. Frigidity can be caused by decreased blood flow to the pelvis. Cancer can be accelerated by decreased blood flow to tissues. When blood flow is decreased to cells in the bone marrow and spleen, it comes full circle and the immune system is weakened.

There is a way to deal with arteriosclerosis. The answer is "natural chelation" based on acidic chelating agents and oxidants that work in concert with other essential nutrients found only in a raw fruit and vegetable diet to reverse plaques and blockages. You would use a safe product to remove the sludge from the pipes in your home, so why not use raw fruits and vegetables to clean your own arteries and organs? When you take control of what you ingest, you likely won't have to call on a cardiologist or a vascular specialist to help clean out the sludge.

Chapter 15

Plantarian Lifestyle for the Family

It's time for another rousing lesson forged in truth along with some sage advice about eating raw fruits and vegetables as a family. After all, what's good for the parents is great for the children.

In 2009, the American Dietetic Association reported that properly planned vegetarian diets, which include total vegetarian or vegan diets, are healthy, provide adequate nutrition, and may also aid in the prevention and treatment of specific diseases (Craig & Mangels, 2009). Such diets are suitable for people of all ages. They are suitable during pregnancy, while breast feeding, and during infancy, childhood, adolescence, and are even good for athletes (Craig & Mangels, 2009).

The Association also noted that, based on reviewed evidence, vegetarian diets that exclude tofu and soy byproducts reduce the risk of death from ischemic heart disease, reduce low-density lipoprotein cholesterol levels, lower blood pressure, and reduce rates of hypertension and Type II diabetes when compared to non-vegetarians (Craig & Mangels, 2009). The evidence also revealed that vegetarians are inclined to have "a lower body mass index and lower overall cancer rates" because of reduced intake of saturated fat and cholesterol and increased consumption of fruits and vegetables. The latter, eating fruits and veggies, vitamins C and E, carotenoids, and phytochemicals that lower serum homocysteine levels (Craig & Mangels, 2009).

Total serum cholesterol and low-density lipoprotein cholesterol levels are usually lower in vegetarians due to decreased damage to the cells and DNA, but high-density lipoprotein cholesterol and triglyceride levels vary depending on the type of vegetarian diet that is followed. True vegetarians adhere to raw foods and do not consume meat and/or dairy substitutes or supplementation that tends to reduce the incidence of hypertension when compared to non-vegetarians. This effect appears to be independent of both body weight and sodium intake. Type II diabetes is less likely to cause death in vegetarians than non-vegetarians, perhaps because of their higher intake of complex carbohydrates (King, 2014).

The occurrence of lung and colorectal cancers are also lower in vegetarians than in non-vegetarians. Reduced colorectal cancer risk is associated with increased consumption of raw fiber, vegetables, and fruit (Chapman, 2014). The environment of the colon is notably different in vegetarians, which may be why they have a lower risk for colon cancer compared to non-vegetarians. Further, breast cancer rates are considerably lower in China, where a plant-based diet is predominant. On the other hand, Japaneses women who consume meat-based diets similar to Western-style diets have an eight times greater chance of developing breast cancer (Vegetarian Foods, n.d.).

Meat and dairy products have been connected to many forms of cancer, including cancer of the colon, breasts, ovaries, and prostate. It's important to note that vegetarian diets must not include processed vegetarian foods in order for the cancer risk to be lowered. Lower rates of cancer have not been as significant in Western vegetarians, possibly due to high consumption of processed vegetarian foods, such as meat/dairy substitutes and supplementations.

The lower estrogen levels in vegetarian women may be protective. According to John A. McDougall, M.D., a high-fat diet will increase the levels of estrogen, progesterone, and prolactin (hormones in a woman's body) through the application of a range of mechanisms. Certain types of bacteria that normally live in the colon of women who eat fatty foods can convert bile acids into other materials that act like hormones or have hormonal activity (McDougall, 2014). This is basically recirculation of hormones. For example, estrogens that are made in the ovaries and the adrenal glands are secreted into the blood stream and then pass through the liver into the intestines. To prevent re-absorption by the intestines, those estrogens are combined in the liver with a non-absorbable substance (McDougall, 2014).

McDougall holds that "Fats, especially meat fats, will encourage the growth of those colon bacteria that are capable of splitting the complexes," which means that"making free-estrogens available for re-absorption can contribute to a situation that favors development of breast cancer" (2014). The fibers in vegetable foods play a strong hand in stopping the absorption of the "free" estrogens that can be found in the bowel, which is why women on vegetarian diets "excrete two to three times more estrogen in their bowel movements, and their blood levels of specific powerful estrogens are 50 percent lower when compared to non-vegetarian women (McDougall, 2014).

A well-planned vegetarian diet may also help prevent and treat renal disease. According to the Academy of Nutrition and Dietetics, research revealed that a plant-based diet may slow down some of the complications associated with chronic kidney disease "such as heart disease, protein loss in urine and the progression of kidney damage" (2010). Studies using human and animal models suggest that some plant proteins may increase survival rates and decrease proteinuria, glomerular filtration rate (the flow rate of filtered fluid through the kidney), renal blood flow, and histologic renal damage compared with a non-vegetarian diet (Chronic, n.d.).

Life Lesson—Karen's Dad

Karen, an R.N in the surgical department, wrote to thank me for "motivating my dad to improve his health." Her father was diagnosed with prostate cancer one year earlier at age 57 and decided to follow my nutritional recommendations. Jean told me, "Since January 2005, he lost 30 pounds in just 30 days . . . he now feels better, sleeps better, has increased energy, and I know he has reduced his prostate cancer progression." She was also motivated to change her own eating habits.

Changing or Establishing Good Eating Habits

Eating habits develop in early childhood. Cooked sources of protein and carbohydrates should not exceed five percent of the diet for children and teens. Choosing a 95 percent plantarian diet can give your child—and your whole family—the opportunity to learn to enjoy a variety of wonderful, nutritious foods.

Children who grow up eating fruits and vegetables are generally slimmer and healthier, and live longer than their carnivorous friends. It is much healthier to build a nutritious diet from plant foods than from animal products. Plant foods provide a healthier source of carbohydrates, sufficient energy and protein, and other health-promoting nutrients such as antioxidants, fiber, minerals, phytochemicals, and vitamins.

Infants do not need any nourishment other than breast milk for the first half-year of life, and they should continue to receive it at least through their first twelve months. Not only are the infant's nutritional needs best met by mother's breast milk, the baby's immunity and psychological well-being are also supported. If the mother is consuming a raw fruits and vegetable diet, the baby will reap the benefits through her breast milk. However, mothers who breastfeed and consume saturated fats and simple carbohydrates are doing their babies no favors. A mother who consumes bottles of carbonated beverages is actually loading her baby up with bad carbs, and the carbonation will cause severe gas and digestive problems for mother and child.

Interestingly, breast-fed babies grow more slowly than bottle-fed babies. Somewhat less rapid growth during the early years is thought to decrease disease risk later in life (Gillman, 2008). Nature may well have designed the human body to grow slower, reach puberty later, and last longer than it does for those raised on omnivorous diets, which underscores why breast feeding is so good for infants.

At about five to six months of age, or when a baby's weight has doubled, other foods can be added to the diet. A good choice would be raw fruit prepared in a food processor. I have also discovered that mixing fruits and vegetables either as they are or in a food processor adds to palatability. Still, many moms and dads worry about feeding their children a plantarian diet because they fear it will lack protein and calcium. Children do need both to grow. However, since the largest part of the diet comes from a variety of raw fruits and vegetables, the baby will receive more than an adequate level of protein and calcium. Deficiencies are extremely unlikely with such a plentiful combination.

It is true that very young children need a slightly higher fat intake than adults. Healthier fat sources include fresh coconuts and avocados. A small percentage (five percent or less) of a child's diet can be supplied by processed foods on special occasions such as birthdays or holidays, but watch out for the hyperactivity reaction to those foods. The following section has been organized to provide you with flexible age guidelines for the plantarian child and the reasons behind those suggestions. You may find they work well for your baby and for you.

Newborn to One Year

The foundation for a life of wellness is created during the first year of life. The idea is to help children develop healthy bodies, not obese bodies. Solid foods are typically introduced in the middle of the first year. Weaning a child from breast-feeding should be done in small increments utilizing soft plant foods such as mashed fruits and vegetables. Start with vegetables such as potatoes, green beans, carrots and peas. They can be lightly steamed and prepared in a food processor. Then add fresh, uncooked fruits such as bananas, avocados, peaches, and/or apples that have been run through the food processor. Finally, add protein-rich foods starting at around eight months of age, such as raw spinach and broccoli prepared in the food processor.

There are exceptions to light steaming. Food temperature should never rise above 130 degrees. Keep in mind that exposing the raw fruits and vegetables to a temperature greater than 105.6 degrees can and will destroy significant nutrients, including the protein found in root vegetables like carrots, potatoes, sweet potatoes, and rutabaga. Steaming should be temperature controlled and can be done in preparation for food processing.

Children Do Become Teens

It seems that if teens are not causing trouble, they feel troubled, especially when it comes to self-image and weight control. Statistics reveal that children and teens are suffering from a shocking obsession with body image. Being thinner is the number one wish among girls age 11 to 17, and even five-year-old girls are concerned about gaining weight (Body, 2014). In fact, the Council on Size and Weight Discrimination revealed that girls in those age groups are more concerned about becoming fat "than they are of nuclear war, cancer, or losing their parents (Body, 2014). That's pure insanity and something parents and counselors should focus on to help those children caught in the quagmire of weight loss and weight control.

This is how bad things really are. Dieting is totally common among over 90 percent of juniors and seniors in high school, though only 10 to 15 percent have weight problems (Body, 2014). According to the Eating Disorders Association, many teens are at risk for developing eating disorders due to their obsession with weight and body image, which can lead to irregular or no menstruation, skin problems, kidney and liver damage, loss of bone mass, hair loss, infertility, irregular heartbeats, cardiac arrest, and eventually death (Body, 2014). And it's not confined to girls. Approximately one million teenage boys have eating disorders and as many as 400,000 are steroid users (Body, 2014).

There is a counter-balance between self-image and weight control. If young people struggle with weight, they most likely struggle with poor self-image and low self-esteem issues. Everyone wrestles with self-doubt at times, but weight control should not cause youngsters as much heartache as it does. Children need exposure to positive reinforcement, but that doesn't mean disingenuously inflating their egos. It means making provisions for and exposing them to superior, knowledgeable role models and supplying them with facts about lifestyle consequences.

Sadly, many parents have issues with their own weight control, poor health, and self-esteem. Thus the sins of the parents are visited upon the children. For example, in 1997, Dr. Robert C. Whitaker and colleagues showed that "the risk of adult obesity was significantly greater if either the child's mother or father was obese" and that obese parents "more than doubled the risk for children, obese or [non-obese], to become obese adults" (Kral & Faith, 2009, citing Whitaker et al., 1997).

So where do the children and teens look for role models? While programs to improve childhood obesity are growing, more emphasis should be placed on positive role models, not the Hollywood variety. They have their own issues with weight and eating healthy. In fact, many of those "mentors" suffer from obesity or other diet-related ailments. As an example, adult drug use has reached alarming rates, surpassing those of the teens. From 2002 to 2007, illicit drug use jumped 116 percent among Americans age fifty-five to fifty-nine, but dropped among those who are between the ages of twelve and seventeen (Deans, 2008). So in order to confront the health issues plaguing children, adults must first confront their own poor lifestyle choices.

Most children eventually look to others as role models instead of their parents or guardians, which is not uncommon among teens. However, they rarely pick role models who live healthy lifestyles and put wellness ahead of self-glorification. Instead, they choose those who will never help them and who, in fact, generally increase their problems. Those scandalous, celluloid role models boast fame, fortune, and perfect bodies whereby teens, in particular, want to emulate their lifestyles. In fact, those same superficially perfect people are used by well-compensated advertising agencies that spin direct media campaigns to entice teenage consumers to spend their money on the food products they endorse. Fad and packaged food diet ads starring high-profile stars or fabulously fit models deceptively appeal to the young person's sense of self-indulgence and well-being.

It's true that some children who have parents with healthy eating habits and strong self-esteem experience weight management problems. But statistics, which form the basis of my contention, show that those children are few and far between, and the number of children that were not as fortunate is far greater.

Life Lesson—Dedra & Family

Dedra, a Patient Care Technician at the hospital in 2002, took my back safety and wellness class. When she met me six months earlier, she shared the results of her blood work. Some of her lab results were staggering:

Triglycerides—500

Cholesterol—396

Blood Sugar—220

Blood Pressure—167/90

Weight—220 pounds

Her doctor told her if the she didn't do something, she would soon die. This caused her to worry because she had a six-year-old son. Her doctor was going to put her on Lipitor and another medication for her blood sugar. "You encouraged me to change my eating habits and lifestyle instead of taking pills." It took Dedra six months, but her lab results were strikingly different:

Triglycerides—173

Cholesterol—196

Blood Sugar—80

Blood Pressure—117/70

Weight—180

Dedra accomplished all of this without taking any medications, which amazed her doctor. She did low-level exercises daily, had more energy, and could do more with her son. She could get through a workday without feeling tired and, with the help of her father (who got on the healthy lifestyle bandwagon), she was sticking with the program. Ironically, her father lost 50 pounds, which was great for him because he was a heart patient. Her son even became aware at the age of six of how much junk food was served at his school. It started with one mom who wanted to live a life of wellness and it became a family affair.

The Bottom Line

The plantarian lifestyle provides many benefits for children of all ages caught in this vicious cycle. School-aged children don't have to deal with the emotional conflict of taking life to sustain life. Adolescents raised on a plantarian diet often find they have an easy time maintaining a healthy weight and have fewer problems with acne, allergies, and gastrointestinal problems than their meat-eating peers. Providing children with knowledge of the plantarian lifestyle is one of the most important things parents and society as a whole can do.

Another important reason (among many) that teens are suffering from obesity or eating disorders is the propaganda spewed in public and private schools. I've noticed first hand this type of irresponsible teaching in our elite and prestigious high schools, where obesity and diet-related diseases might be at the same disturbing levels as the government-owned public schools.

For example, when the school my son attended invited a registered dietitian to educate the class about healthy eating, she opened up the dialogue by asking the 12-15 class attendees how many of them thought there were good foods and bad foods. Of course my son, who was nutrient-educated by me, and two or three other children raised their hands to agree with the factual statement. The registered dietitian bluntly disagreed with them and said they were all wrong. She had the temerity to add that, "All foods are good to eat." It would have been very difficult for me to believe my son's story if I hadn't seen her handout, which he brought home. It stated just that.

I was surprised that the teacher, who was present, didn't have the security guard toss this alleged registered dietician out of the classroom immediately. This is a classic example of irresponsible teaching that confuses our children who then go on to become bulimic, anorexic, diabetic, hypertensive, and cancer patients down the road, and who will end up going to the same robots to learn how to control their diseases instead of how to prevent and reverse them.

Let me close out this chapter with a story. I once had a meeting with a local physician—an adult internist—from whom I was requesting support to begin a wellness program for unhealthy and obese children. His response to my plan was outrageous. He said that if I improve the health of the teenagers, his business and that of other physicians would drastically suffer due to a shortage of sick adults. His statement vividly resonates throughout the whole healthcare industry. As long as physicians practice with a "keep the people sick and their money coming" mentality, and as long as registered dietitians continue to give false advice, there truly is no hope for the children unless parents take control, stand for what's right, and help their children achieve a state of wellness without interference from the so-called professionals.

Chapter 16

Plant-Based Nutrition for Seniors

There are those in our society who look upon senior citizens as just biding their time before leaving this world. Helping them medically, to some, is a waste of money and precious medical resources. However, today's seniors have plenty of time left to contribute to society, and a healthy diet geared toward wellness is one way to take them off the "useless eaters" list and add them to the "still productive" list.

Making the switch to a plantarian diet is challenging for even the most health-conscious individuals, but a gradual switch makes the change easier to tolerate, without hunger and cravings. Seniors need to make an extra-conscious effort to embrace this lifestyle change. Years of eating processed foods takes a toll by producing numerous health issues that society almost always blames on aging. While aging does cause natural changes in appearance and hormone levels, many common complaints, syndromes, illnesses, and diseases can be avoided through a plantarian lifestyle.

Aging bodies undergo a series of nutrient depletions. Enzymes, minerals, and vitamins are needed to fuel metabolism and constantly repair damaged cells. It is essential to supply the body with highly dense nutrients from raw fruits and vegetables to prevent complete nutrient depletion and the breakdown of muscle mass. Nutrient depletion in senior citizens also speeds up the vicious cycle of induced toxicity that taxes the immune systems, diminishes the ability to fight disease, and starts a chain or chains of events that can and often do show up on the heels of a disease or illness. The following illustrates how changing the diet of one senior citizen affected her senior citizen daughter and her doctor. It's really a story about a miracle.

Life Lesson—Marjorie, Her Daughter & Her Doctor

This was a triple play, all of which focused on a 92-year-old woman's journey to wellness and the results of that journey. At age 92, Marjorie was resigned to the fact that nothing could improve her quality of life due to various physical problems. However, she was wrong because, as she wrote, ". . . your program of dietary suggestions, along with minimum exercises, has really helped the quality of my life." Marjorie lost almost 70 pounds, had a marked decrease in the swelling of her legs, and was no longer on Lasix. Her balance improved, as did her walking, the pain in her shoulder decreased, and she had more energy.

"I am actually able to assist and participate in different projects and activities in my community." Six months earlier, Marjorie was taking 11 different medications daily, but her doctor, P.R., M.D., was amazed by her progress: "By following your dietary instructions and minimum exercises, she has improved her overall health ... reduced her chronic joint pains . . . and was more active and sociable during her recent visit. I have been able to reduce her prescription medications to a minimum (three or four as needed)."

Her daughter, Nancy, wrote, "Before you came into her life she had almost given up. She had a difficult time getting around and could hardly use her right arm and shoulder. She weighed 220 pounds, used a rolling walker and still had frequent falls." After receiving physical therapy from me and following my nutritional recommendations, Marjorie walked without a walker, had less joint pain, almost no falls for six months, and her weight was down to 150 pounds. Her daughter wrote, "She used to stay in her own apartment most of the time; now she goes to restaurants and participates in social life at [her senior community]." For Marjorie's daughter, such vast improvements gave her a sense of well-being about her mother and something she could also do for herself that would add years to her own life.

The following guidelines can help reverse the downside of aging in seniors who have always consumed processed foods and now want to adapt to a plantarian lifestyle. These guidelines also work well for younger people who want to prevent depletion of energy and vitamins due to aging. The steps are gradual to help each person adapt to and tolerate the plantarian lifestyle without shocking the body.

Step One

Clear out old accumulations from the intestinal tract. This can be accomplished by a gradual shift away from processed foods. Eat two or three apples for breakfast. Eating an apple prior to every meal provides proper nutrients and is high in fiber (which promotes digestion), and its complexity will encourage you to eat less cooked foods at mealtime. Most complex colon-cleansing procedures include whole apples or derivatives like apple sauce, because apples are a powerful cleansing food (Huff, 2013). Apples are also rich in a carbohydrate compound called pectin, which operates as a thickening agent in the digestive tract. When pectin is taken in therapeutic doses it "helps root out built-up toxins in the colon and strengthen the intestinal lining" (Huff, 2013). Other fruits may be used, but my favorite is the apple.

Eat a good-size garden salad that includes broccoli, cauliflower, cucumber, onions, spinach, and tomatoes prior to your mid-day and evening meals. Limit dressing to lime juice and/or vinegar. This will help you feel full and avoid gorging on unhealthy foods when eating your main meal. Eventually, work on doing away with all dressing so you can enjoy the true taste of the vegetables.

If you must snack during the day, snack on raw fruits and vegetables. The human body craves fruits and vegetables more than almost any other food because we don't eat enough of them to meet our nutritional needs (Bollinger, 2012). There was a time when we thought two or three servings of fruits and veggies (or even less) was sufficient, but the Centers for Disease Control and Prevention (CDC) and the USDA both recommend a minimum of five servings per day (Bollinger, 2012). Bollinger writes, "What you're missing could be the difference between just surviving and all-out thriving" (2012). It's never too late to start down this healthy road to wellness. All it takes is some creative thinking, proper planning, and a small amount of effort to make snacking far more nutritious.

Limit portions of cooked, processed food to one meal a day and approximately five percent of the total daily food intake, with servings no larger than a fist. Eat generous portions of raw vegetables as side dishes. Reserve cooked food consumption for the most tempting time of day. Your goal is to choose natural, raw fruits and vegetables as often as you can, and only go with processed foods if you're in a bind. As Christine Richmond noted in *23 Ways to Eat Clean*, "Here, we show how common foods morph from real (i.e. apples) to highly processed (apple toaster pastries)" (2014). It's better to stay away from morphed foods.

Case in point: Back in the 1970s, a Chiffon margarine television commercial aired repeatedly to sell us fake butter. It featured Dena Dietrich, a mom type portraying the mythical Mother Nature. When I think of all the processed foods out there, that commercial, available on YouTube.com, comes to mind because her infamous line was, "It's not nice to fool Mother Nature." (2010). Well, that's what processed foods are doing, but they can't fool your body because your body knows the truth.

Step Two

To be well-nourished means to provide the body with everything it requires for cellular nutrition and immune system enzyme replenishment. It also means complete elimination of all the resultant debris, which includes having bowel movements two to three times daily. Think of nutrition, enzyme replacement, and waste elimination as the building blocks of wellness and longevity, and don't be victimized by self-delusion. Digestive symptoms go undiagnosed as a result of denial. Manifested conditions like belching, bloating, constipation, diarrhea, flatulence, food sensitivities, gas, indigestion, irritable bowel syndrome (IBS), and malabsorption are common conditions that are considered normal. They're not. Something as innocuous as a sluggish bowel can harbor pounds of unprocessed toxic fecal matter. The average American carries approximately sixteen pounds of fecal matter in his/her intestinal tract daily. That's enough to make you as irritable and sluggish as your equally irritable and sluggish intestinal tract (Gates, 2014).

According to Dr. Lynn Hardy, N.D., C.N.C., self-poisoning from a sluggish digestive tract affects all the cells in our bodies. If toxins build up in the nervous system, the result is irritability and depression. And if those toxins back up into the heart, we experience weakness (1999-2003). If they head to the stomach, we feel bloated, and when they reach the lungs, our breath is atrocious (Hardy, 1999-2003). When those poisons use the skin as their escape route, we develop rashes and blotches, look pale, and the skin looks wrinkled (Hardy, 1999-2003). Finally, if those toxins invade the glands, "we feel fatigued, lethargic, our sex drive may cease and we appear to look much older than our actual age" (Hardy, 1999-2003).

If eating results in bloating, gas, or occasional abdominal pains, consider digestive enzymes. Taking enzymes at the beginning of each meal from raw food sources optimizes digestion, increases nutrition, strengthens the ability to fight off disease, replenishes immune system enzymes, and decreases exposure to antigens—food particles that can stimulate allergic reactions. Often, a SAD diet leads to dehydration, which leads to chronic constipation and, over a number of years, results in a condition called diverticulitis, defined as a weakness of the muscle layer in the colon wall.

When the typical person rests in a chair or lies down, 25 percent of the body's available energy goes toward maintaining digestive health. During and immediately after food consumption, incrementally higher levels of energy depletion occur. By consuming enzymes from raw food sources, less energy goes toward digestion, leaving more available to make repairs, restore normal functions, and maintain or rebuild vitality. Falling asleep after a meal is the body's natural way of conserving energy for digestion. This sleep phenomenon is a huge indicator of a body that lacks nourishment and suffers serious physiological stress. It also indicates a sudden blood sugar plummet following a highly processed meal.

It's never too late to improve your digestive system. The human body, regardless of age or condition, has an incredible capacity to heal and repair itself. Two weeks after following these recommendations, bowel movements should occur more frequently and digestion will cause less stress.

Life Lesson—Jo & Richard

Jo was an attendee at a senior citizen residential center wellness program I conducted. When she moved to the center she was "very healthy, vigorous, and active." Six years later, at age 88, she was "lethargic, lazy, and sleepy most of the time." She stated that it was because everything was done for the residents of the center. They didn't have to cook, wash dishes, wash sheets and towels, or even clean their apartments. They didn't have to drive themselves to the stores, their doctors, or even to go sightseeing. All that was left for them to do was take a nap.

Jo was a woman who used to walk half a mile everyday, but all she could do before my presentation was walk to the dining room for meals. Then everything changed. "After three weeks of eating [a plantarian diet] and exercising . . . I feel like a new person." Jo was eating lots of apples and other raw fruits and vegetables. It made a huge difference in her life.

Richard was also part of the senior citizen residential center program I taught to help improve the quality of elderly lives. "I have been in the program for three weeks, have already experienced multiple benefits from it, and expect to gain even more as I continue. I sincerely hope that James will be able to continue to provide these benefits to any resident that wants to achieve a better lifestyle."

Step Three

Most seniors have a lot of interaction with doctors. Holding doctors accountable for answering questions and giving full explanations about treatment only makes sense and ensures that the patient receives the care he/she needs. Patients benefit from asking questions, and they should not be put off by rude doctors who only answer by saying they know best or that they are too busy to answer. If they are too busy to address health concerns, they shouldn't be doctors—yours or anyone else's. Be sure to have a family member or an advocate by your side when visiting your doctor. This will ensure accountability.

Patients should ask whether minor lifestyle changes might help eliminate the need for some drugs. Do not settle for the "this is part of the aging process" answer. Doctors are also fond of saying that certain diseases come from genes, but most diseases don't run in the family. Lifestyle is the catalyst, and diseases correspond with lifestyle. Genes are designed to protect people, not create diseases. They determine certain predispositions, which determine our diseases based on the type of lifestyle we adopt.

One of the most ridiculous processes to occur in a doctor's office is the rigorous family medical history inquiry. My parents' health is not relevant to my current health status. The questions should be rephrased to read: "What are/were your parents' dietary habits? Were you raised by your parents? Do you eat the same foods as your parents? What are your parents' diseases?" Based on the answers, a qualified doctor should be able to predict the type of current and possible future diseases with 90 percent accuracy. Of course, in my opinion, diseases may no longer be determined or controlled by our parents' lifestyles. FDA-approved foods, pharmaceuticals, and unqualified medical professionals are to blame for reprogramming us through deceptive and unconscionable advertising. It's up to us to hunt for the truth.

Remember, no patient should ever fear questioning a doctor. In her article, *Don't be afraid to speak honestly with your doctor*, Dr. Lisa Masterson cited the oft-used cliché, "'What you don't know can't hurt you,'" and stated that such a belief might prove dangerous to the patient (2013). It is her contention that what we don't know might just kill us, which means we must talk with doctors openly and honestly, and ask as many questions as possible to create a foundation for good health (Masterson, 2013).

If your doctor really wants to help, diagnose, treat, and offer you medical advice, make sure you take responsibility for the communication aspect of your health care. It will benefit both you and your doctor, and save precious time and money avoiding rabbit trails that don't need to be followed. This advice includes self-education in wellness and being bold enough to tell your doctor when diet, not medication, is the answer to health problem. Stand up for what you know and believe, even if your doctor doesn't agree with you.

Chapter 17

Energy—How to "Bottle It!"

We've all had days when we feel as though we have one teaspoon of energy left before finally getting into bed for the night. Those of us who are old enough will recall the grape juice commercial that talked about "The Valley of Fatigue," which hit at around 2-3 p.m. every day. Of course, there's that oft-recited lament, "I have no energy left; you deal with it!"

Several years ago I began randomly asking my 80 or 90-year-old patients one question—would you like to be 25 years old again? Almost 100 percent of them replied with a stern, "No!" However, almost 100 percent of them stated "I wish I had the energy I had when I was 25." Approximately three years ago, when I was 50, I was walking alongside one of my 95-year-old patients at a retirement residence. We came upon an eight-year-old girl who was playing with a couple of her friends, jumping around and just being a kid. The 95-year-old woman stopped to watch her play for a few minutes, then looked at me and said, "If only you could bottle up that energy."

I realized that at age 50 I could match or surpass the little girl's energy level. I have always been envied by friends and co-workers for my high energy levels, and have even been accused of being on some kind of energy-boosting supplement, drink, or drug. Although I don't have the secret to the legendary Fountain of Youth (because I have gotten older over the years), I do believe that I've been able to bottle up the energy that everyone covets, even those in their early thirties, and I don't need energy boosting supplements, drinks, or drugs to create false energy.

Life Lesson—Nancy Wants My Energy

Nancy was a 9th floor nurse who wrote that I often had to "hop over a walker or do a pull up on an overhead trapeze just to provide inspiration" to the patients. I wanted the patients and my co-workers to quit smoking, make diet modifications to lose excess weight, and be active. "James is a walking (or running!) billboard. He lives what he 'preaches,' [and] he exemplifies our purpose statement to improve the health of the people we touch." Nancy believed I touched lives by teaching back safety, working as a physical therapist assistant, and offering "words of personal encouragement for those who are trying to 'work' his program." That program always included suggestions about healthy eating the plantarian way. It's the foundation for any journey to wellness.

Energy Defined

So, what is energy? What is it that makes us feel superhuman one minute and like the "last rose of summer" the next? A simple definition would read something like—energy is the strength and vigor required for continuous physical and/or mental activity. Yes, even your brain needs energy to carry out its various functions, including thinking and daydreaming. However, now that we know what energy really is, where does it come from, and how do we get some so we're not just limping through life? The answer is found in the consumption of all those delicious raw fruits and vegetables.

As the human body ages, it's not as forgiving and it becomes imperative to consume more digestible foods for greater energy. Foods that contain the right nutrients in the right balance require less essential nutrients from the body for the digestion process. When we consume ingestible substances that are depleted of enzymes and micro and macronutrients, the body has to work harder to digest those substances, which leads to more depletion of essential nutrients. Continued depletion of those nutrients used up while the body works to digest indigestible substances makes us vulnerable to common colds, viruses, and other ailments. And if we continue to ingest indigestible substances, we may wind up with more serious diseases. This process also robs us of our daily energy.

According to the folks at Ask.com, human beings "get energy by releasing the stored chemical energy in the foods they eat," and those foods are comprised of different kinds of macromolecules, each one holding a different amount of energy (2014). After we eat, the food we've ingested is broken down via catabolic metabolism to fuel all of our biological functions. Think of a fire that is burning brightly. It takes oxygen to make that fire in the first place and for it to continue burning. The same applies to the way we burn food for energy. It's called aerobic metabolism, which must have oxygen to burn food and explains why we need oxygen to live (ask.com, 2014). If our exercise level is too intense, the body will switch to anaerobic metabolism, which produces unwanted waste products such as lactic acid—one of the chemicals that exacerbates chronic pain.

There are, unfortunately, situations, concerns, states of mind and body, and other internal and external forces that suppress our energy levels. Once you understand what some of them are and how they rob you of your precious energy, you will be able to control them, overcome them, and eventually reach a state of homeostasis.

The Impact of Chronic Pain

Chronic pain is an energy suppressant. The general consensus on chronic pain is that it lasts longer than 12 weeks; however, others define it as any pain that lasts more than six months. Whereas acute pain is a normal sensation that alerts us to possible injury, chronic pain is very different because it persists. According to WebMD, approximately 100 million Americans experience chronic pain, which can be mild, come in spurts (episodic), be continuous, excruciating, simply annoying, or it can totally incapacitate the sufferer (2014). The pain signals in your body can stay active for weeks, months, or years and affect most people emotionally as well as physically.

Many people endure chronic headaches, joint pain, pain from injury, and backaches. Others suffer from tendon inflammations (tendinitis), sinus inflammations (sinusitis), the traveling effects of carpal tunnel syndrome, and other pain that finds a home in definitive body parts such as one or both shoulders, the neck, or the pelvis. It can also include pain in the muscles and/or nerves. Chronic pain can be the result of an injury or infection, but it can also occur absent of any injury or damage to the body. The main cause of premature aging, which leads to degenerative changes and chronic pain, is the moderate or regular consumption of indigestible substances resulting in poor circulation or lack of sufficient nutrients in the blood.

Some causes of chronic pain are due to years of abuse to the body, such as decades of poor posture, lifting and carrying heavy objects improperly, obesity, regular jogging, smoking and its effects on the back and knees, scoliosis (a congenital condition also called curvature of the spine), wearing high heels, and/or sleeping on a low-support mattress. Let's face it, a great deal of energy is expended dealing with chronic pain, which includes emotional expenditures such as stress, depression, anxiety, anger, and fatigue—all of which suppress the body's immune system, the body's natural painkillers (endorphins), and likely increase chemicals that increase pain. By the time you've reached that point in your chronic pain existence, you're ready to throw in the towel. However, there are edible solutions that come in the form of raw fruits and vegetables, all of which help defeat chronic pain.

For example, cherries contain a compound called anthocyanin that works in two ways to tamp down pain. Anthocyanin blocks inflammation and inhibits pain enzymes. Ginger works like a natural aspirin to alleviate pain and inflammation and is often used to calm an upset stomach, stop nausea, and even helps with seasickness. It seems to rid the gut of intestinal gas and block a receptor in the stomach that brings on vomiting. This little wonder root also offers relief from migraines, arthritis pain, and muscle aches.

The Impact of Stress

Stress is a state of mental or emotional strain or tension caused by difficult or very demanding situations from either external (in one's surroundings) or physiological (internal) sources. Stressful events might be part of our daily living, but they cause an increase in our cortisol levels, which causes food cravings (Glassman, 2014). If we are brought up on high fat, salt, and sugary foods, we will crave those types of foods during stressful or happy times. Food cravings are the result of taste buds' memory and how that memory connects us to our past and our upbringing. We have the power to retrain our taste buds by introducing more plant foods into our diets to create new memories and cravings. It is imperative that the body be armed with a strong line of defense and a strong immune system in order to survive such environmental stressors.

There are a multitude of stress-producing situations that occur throughout our lives such as moving from one home to another—this is especially stressful when moving to another geographical location. The death of a spouse, family member, friend, or even acquaintance is a serious stress producer. Pregnancy also produces stress, as do injury, illness, and being the victim of a crime—i.e., sexual molestation, mugging, assault, or burglary. Drug and alcohol abuse are traditional escape routes used by those who are overstressed. However, in using drugs or drinking alcohol, the abuser has added to the stress his/her body is already experiencing. It takes a lot of physical energy to cope with such a chemical assault on the body.

Changes in the family unit as a result of marriage and/or the addition of a new baby are extremely stressful, as are separation and divorce. Add to that the rise in sexual problems and infirmities, and the stress meter hits the red zone. Of course, the worst stress we put on our bodies is caused by the moderate or regular consumption of processed foods that lack the nutrients our bodies need to cope with stress, be healthy, and achieve wellness.

Asparagus supposedly makes urine smell funky, but it's high in folate, which is needed to maintain calmness and contains serotonin, a mood stabilizer (Fight Stress, 2014). Avocados literally stress-proof the body because they're high in glutathione, which blocks the intestinal absorption of specific fats that cause cell damage. They also contain lutein, beta-carotene, vitamin E, and loads of B vitamins (Glassman, 2014).

Bananas contain potassium, a vital mineral for keeping blood pressure low, while oranges and berries such as strawberries, raspberries, and blackberries are high in vitamin C, which helps combat stress. In fact, blueberries contain extremely high levels of the antioxidant anthocyanin (Glassman, 2014). Swiss chard is high in magnesium and, like other leafy greens, helps balance cortisol, the body's stress hormone, and spinach contains magnesium, which helps improve your body's response to stress and may prevent migraine headaches (Fight Stress, 2014). Finally, carrots are nutrient rich and they're crunchy—something you can sink your teeth into to beat stress.

If you're stressed, do yourself a favor and avoid consuming substances that will only make things worse. Caffeine, which is in coffee, soda, tea, and chocolate, among other beverages and alleged foods, will definitely raise all stress hormone levels. Sugar (simple carbohydrates) causes sudden increases in blood glucose levels, increases insulin output, and negatively affects the adrenal glands that normalize stress hormones and aid the thyroid in regulating body weight (Fight Stress, 2014).

Trans-fatty acids, or trans-fats, found in all hydrogenated vegetable oils, are used in most cakes, cookies, and breads. They can harm the immune system and increase the risk of heart disease (Fight Stress, 2014). Finally, excessive alcohol consumption puts additional sugar in the body, which can damage the adrenal glands and can lead to liver damage and diabetes (Fight Stress, 2014).

The Impact of Anxiety/Worrying

We all know what it feels like to worry, be nervous, or experience unease (think dis-ease). Usually, such a state of being revolves around something that's about to happen, or something that has an unknown or uncertain outcome. Anxiety disorders can be the result of problems in our living, work, or even educational environments. Medical factors, genetics, brain chemistry, substance abuse, or any combination of these are also contributors to anxiety and worry. Anxiety and/or worrying are most commonly set off by stress in our lives. It is extremely common for anxiety to be a response to outside forces, but it is equally possible that we make ourselves anxious by thinking or talking in the negative or by telling ourselves that whatever can go wrong will go wrong. As with the causes of stress, trauma can result from abuse, being the victim of a crime, the death of loved ones, upheavals in personal relationships (marriages or friendships), stress at work or school, stress about finances/money, an impending divorce, the results of a natural disaster, or even something like oxygen deprivation in high-altitude regions.

Whatever the cause, the solution is to use diet to achieve balance, clear thinking, and overall wellness. Eating raw fruits and vegetables, as we've already discussed in the previous sections of this chapter, will increase your ability to not just cope with anxiety and worry, but to eliminate them completely. Start with a good breakfast to maintain healthy blood sugar levels during the day. This will help reduce stress and anxiety. Eat small meals and munch on healthy snacks throughout the day, avoid consuming processed foods, and steer clear of coffee and other caffeinated drinks (Shaw, 2010). They will only make you more anxious and drinking them will adversely affect your ability to sleep.

Studies have demonstrated the relationship between the B vitamins and mood, which includes thiamin or vitamin B1 (Orenstein, 2014). Some people suffer from depression from a B12 and folic acid deficiency, which makes it wise to eat foods rich in B vitamins to prevent anxiety—leafy greens, oranges and other citrus fruits (Orenstein, 2014).

The Impact of Sleep Deprivation and Deficiency

Sleep deprivation, or not getting enough sleep, is linked to many chronic health problems and is often caused by the moderate or regular ingestion of the indigestible substances we call food. Those chronic health problems include, but are not limited to, heart disease, kidney disease, high blood pressure, diabetes, stroke, obesity, and depression. An article in *Fitness Magazine* by Ana Mantica told the story of an active 34-year-old woman who played league soccer but was tired all the time (2014). After discussing her fatigue and lack of energy with a teammate, she realized that her diet was contributing to her sleepless nights (Mantica, 2014). She got rid of the alcohol and caffeine, cut out consumption of snacks loaded with sugar, started eating fruits and vegetables, and within just a few days, she started feeling better. Changing her diet meant she slept better and longer, woke up refreshed, and had more energy and stamina at work and while playing soccer (Mantica, 2014).

When the body is in physiological harmony, it can comfortably and efficiently function on five to six hours of asleep. This is in stark contrast to those who consume processed foods during the day, stay in bed an average of eight or nine hours, toss and turn throughout the night, and wind up with only three or four hours of sleep. They are the same individuals who complain of day-time fatigue and poor energy levels, consume energy drinks and supplements, and finally resort to sleeping pills, which ultimately mask the real and very serious causes of sleep disorders and deprivation.

Foods that are high in magnesium and potassium found in many vegetables and fruits contribute to improved circulation and help body muscles relax (Breus, 2013). Researchers have discovered that your potassium-regulating mechanism may help produce the deepest sleep phase (short-wave sleep), and foods high in calcium help in the production of the hormone melatonin, which is needed to generate slow-wave sleep. Those same foods also help preserve a proper cycle of sleeping and waking (Breus, 2013).

Foods that help your body produce a healthy sleep cycle include such tasty treats as cherries, especially tart cherries, which help increase melatonin levels.

Leafy greens such as kale are loaded with calcium, which helps the brain make use of tryptophan to produce melatonin. Conversely, foods that have little or no nutritional value are often high in substances that will keep you awake—bad fats, sugar, salt, caffeine, and empty calories.

Life Lesson—Carol's Journey to Wellness

Carol was a Patient Care Technician in 2002 at the hospital. She attended my back safety and wellness class and, after following my recommendations, wrote to tell me about the impact it had on her life after just three weeks. She wrote, "My back no longer hurts; my feet don't hurt, my legs don't hurt and are no longer tired. I have energy I didn't have before. I am not tired, I don't need as much sleep. I walk about three times a week. I don't feel sick to my stomach after I eat a meal. I have lost over 10 pounds and also in inches. Most of all, I am starting to feel good about myself." Carol also noted she was drinking some water, and her skin felt better because it was moist and not dried out. She, too, was eating to live, not living to eat. "I want to do things now and be a part of life, not just sit and watch life pass me by. I just can't tell you how much energy I have—I feel great!"

Since eating a plantarian diet means consuming all the nutrients you need to achieve wellness, you will also find yourself sleeping better, enjoying 2-3 additional hours in your day because you don't require as much sleep, and you will be filled with the kind of energy that allows you to be more productive. Give it a try; you have nothing to lose except a dress or pant size and everything to gain in the way of nights filled with sound sleep. Carol did and look how much it helped her to "feel great."

Chapter 18

The Supplement Scam

Taking vitamins and other nutritional supplements is a modern-day form of quackery. Vitamin manufacturers are making billions of dollars by piggybacking their merchandise on a conditioned consumer response. Everyone wants a "magic bullet" to feel healthy, but those who believe that taking prescribed antibiotics in pill form can cure diseases want the same results from vitamin and mineral supplements. It doesn't work that way.

Let's use a domestic pet example to prove my point. Allegedly, and most likely, dog and cat food kibble has had the nutritional life kicked out of it via the cooking process. Your pet suffers from skin rashes, hair loss, itching, ear infections, and one or more allergies—and the vet bills are piling up while the dog or cat is no better than he/she was prior to taking all those veterinary medicines. Then, while driving in your car, at work, or doing things around the house, you hear an advertisement on the radio for a product that will cure your pet's ills. For well over $100 per month, you can give your pet this magic bullet and he/she will be fine. What's wrong with this picture? Assuming you pay good money for your pet's food, why are you now paying even more money to make up for what that food doesn't do and the harm it's causing? How about changing your pet's diet before investing in what he/she doesn't need?

This is what the same or similar industry is doing to you—shifting the paradigm away from non-nutritious foods to the need to supplement what's not good for you in the first place. Millions of people are taking mega-doses of vitamins, even though their effectiveness has not been scientifically substantiated—it's a quantum leap in logic propelled by the illusion of promised health and longevity. It would be one thing if vitamins consisted of only good ingredients that justified the money spent on them, but it isn't even clear what's in them. What we do know is that they're we do know they're not all that helpful and some actually cause harm.

Carrie Gann, ABC News Medical Unit, reported on a study published in October 2011 in the *Archives of Internal Medicine.* Researchers studied over 38,000 women who were age 55 and older and had also been participants in the *Iowa Women's Health Study* starting in the mid-1980s (Gann, 2011). The study revealed that most supplements had no effect on a woman's health, and those who took specific supplements, such as vitamin B6, folic acid, magnesium, zinc, copper, iron, and multivitamins, might have a slightly higher risk of death than women who did not take those supplements. The only supplement that helped reduce the risk of death was calcium (Gann, 2011).

Notwithstanding evidence against supplementation, the National Institutes of Health (NIH) noted over a decade ago that approximately 50 percent of Americans stated they took at least one dietary supplement, which created almost $20 billion in yearly profits for the industry (Gann, 2011). This increase in use grows exponentially as people get older, i.e., "the numbers of women who reported taking supplements increased over time—from 63 percent in 1986, to 75 percent in 1997 and 85 percent in 2004" (Gann, 2011).

Two days after the study reported by ABC news was released, researchers at the Cleveland Clinic discovered that men who took vitamin E had a higher risk of prostate cancer. But that "discover" supported the findings of seven previous studies that had clearly shown that vitamins increased the risk of cancer, heart disease, and shortened lives (Offit, 2013).

Was the public convinced? Not a chance! In 2012 over 50 percent of all Americans ingested one vitamin supplement or another (Offit, 2013). A report released in 2014 by the U.S. Preventative Services Task Force comprised of an "influential government panel of experts" stated that Americans who are healthy should not take vitamin E or beta carotene supplements to help prevent heart disease or cancer, adding that taking beta carotene might increase health risks not decrease them (Goodman, 2014).

While one might wonder what their definition of healthy is, they also revealed that evidence proves that vitamin E does nothing to prevent heart disease or cancer, and beta carotene may heighten the risk of lung cancer in those already at higher risk for the disease—"on average, extra beta carotene increased the risk of lung cancer in smokers by about 24 percent," (Goodman, 2014).

In order to help guide American consumers, the panel thoroughly examined all studies on vitamins over the past decade—five on multivitamins and 24 on single or paired supplements (Goodman, 2014). Of those studies examined, three out of five found no benefits derived from taking multivitamins, and only two showed that multivitamin intake might cause a slight reduction in the risk of cancer in men who are older (Goodman, 2014).

While representatives from the vitamin/supplement industry did their usual damage control so as not to lose billions of dollars in profits, it's clear that the report proves that one cannot use supplements instead of eating a healthy diet and controlling body weight. As Alice Lichtenstein, professor of nutrition science and policy at Tufts University in Boston, stated, "'The current U.S. Preventive Services Task Force report has collated the available data and confirmed what many of us have suspected—popping a pill is no substitute for eating sensibly and moving more'"(Goodman, 2014).

Another study found that excessive consumption of vitamin A promoted hip fractures in postmenopausal women and birth defects when taken during pregnancy (Feskanich, 2002; Brody 1995). Calcium promoted to prevent osteoporosis in women over sixty years placed them at a higher risk for kidney stones. Excessive amounts of calcium have been shown to promote decreased oxygen flow to the brain (dementia), compromising the ability to perceive reality and reason accordingly (Bakalar, 2013). Though not yet scientifically verified, calcium deposition in all probability is related to its insolubility at low temperatures.

Life Lesson—Donna and Her Supplements

I met Donna while I was providing physical therapy for her bedridden mother and shared my dietary plan with her to help her lose weight. She didn't believe me, though she was spending around $700 per month at a popular nutrition store in town on all kinds of supplements to help her lose weight. She was also going to the gym every day at an additional cost, which I told her not to do. Frustrated by the lack of results, she decided to give my suggestions a try so she could prove me wrong. "He guaranteed I'd lose weight, but I'd been on every diet on the planet two or three times and nothing worked, so I figured what was one more disappointment." Donna lost 10 pounds the first week she was on the plantarian diet and a total of 60 pounds in four months. "I felt wonderful. I always had lots of energy, but now I had more, was sleeping better, and had no indigestion. I was able to stop my blood pressure medicines and was no longer pre-diabetic." On top of that, she had all that extra money to spend on fresh fruits and vegetables instead of supplements that did nothing to improve her health or help her lose weight. Instead of spending time and money at the gym, I told Donna to just stay active. Today, Donna's story should be posted on the walls of every doctor's office and health food store. She's a poster child for why we don't need supplements. What we do need are real and natural nutrients from raw fruits and vegetables, not something locked up in a pill.

Consuming the Real Thing

Real vitamins grow in gardens and on trees. They are not found in pills sold at drug or health food stores. Manufactured supplements cannot reproduce absorption of vitamins in the same manner the body extracts it from raw, natural foods. The essential nutrients found in foods are beneficial to the body only if consumed when they are still in their raw, whole, and natural state. A properly constituted diet that is dominated by raw fruits and vegetables will meet the body's requirements for vitamin nutrition without any artificial augmentation.

Furthermore, large doses of self-prescribed vitamins can alter normal body alkalinity, creating unknown reactions with foods and medicines that can have serious consequences. This doesn't happen if raw fruits and vegetables are the sources of vitamin intake. Even worse, parents who rely on supplements do their children a real disservice, which makes manufacturers of all those sugar-filled cereals exceedingly happy as they drop their massive profits into their respective bank accounts. While books cannot always be judged by their covers, those folks found a way to please the parents by labeling their cereal boxes with "fortified with vitamins" so moms and dads can feel better feeding their children overly sweetened grains—as if the nutrients stuffed into those cereals will negate the high sugar content (Dwyer, 2014).

A report from Environmental Working Group, a health advocacy organization located in Washington, D.C., indicates that cereal companies are supplementing their products with adult-level micronutrients, which can be harmful to children (Dwyer, 2014). The report stated that "'more than 10 million American children are getting too much vitamin A; more than 13 million get too much zinc; and nearly 5 million get too much niacin'" (Dwyer, 2014). The consequences are startling—irreparable liver and skeletal damage from too much vitamin A; stomach pains, vomiting, and an impaired immune system from too much zinc; and more liver damage from too much niacin (Dwyer, 2014) (Schmidt, 2014).

Quite frankly, the FDA (Food & Drug Administration) has a lot of explaining to do because the agency does not control the claims made by vitamin supplement companies regarding each product's performance, even though it's supposed to promote and protect public health. According to the FDA, "dietary supplements are not approved by the government for safety and effectiveness before they are marketed" (Dietary, 2014). If the supplement includes an ingredient that is new, the FDA reviews that ingredient for safety, not effectiveness, but it doesn't approve it prior to marketing (Dietary, 2014). The FDA leaves that obligation to the manufacturers and distributors of those supplements before they are marketed, which means they must adhere to minimum quality standards, guarantee they contain no impurities, and their labels are accurate (Dietary, 2014). It is also now up to the manufacturers to report to the FDA all serious negative reactions, events, or illnesses caused by their supplements, and the FDA can remove products from the market if they are deemed unsafe, contaminated, or product claims are false and/or misleading (Dietary, 2014).

This convinces me that no one should rely on the FDA regarding the need for or quality of vitamins and supplements, or how it monitors claims by supplement companies. The FDA leaves a lot of leeway for those companies to make outrageous claims if they use the right language. As a result, the supplement industry is undeterred by science *and* the FDA, or any product claim warnings. What it really comes down to is the denial of health freedom and free speech—and it's almost obscene how the agency and others are on a rampage to stop health freedom in America. Pro-choice is acceptable only when it does not intrude on the dictates of government entities, the medical profession, pharmaceutical companies, and public and private insurance companies.

While many researchers once believed there were benefits from the proper use of supplemental nutrients and vitamins, current research is taking us back to what our parents and grandparents knew was true—nutrients work best for our bodies when they are eaten as food (Abse, 2012). Our obsession with magic bullets and quick, neatly packaged meals may have started during the 1960s and 1970s when astronauts were flying around space eating foods from plastic tubes (Abse, 2012). Back then, everyone dreamed of utopian living. Today, consumers have shifted their utopian ideals to whole and organic foods, but they still believe that it's healthy to take "concentrated, compressed forms of life-enhancing chemicals" to cure physical woes (Abse, 2012).

It would do us well to remember Brian Maxwell, the world-class marathoner and developer of the Power Bar. Maxwell died in 2002 at the age of fifty-one from coronary artery disease. In 1996, he and his wife, Jennifer, co-founded Power Bar and started selling their energy-boosting confection out of their own kitchen. Over the next ten years, the Berkeley Company reached $150 million in sales and had 300 employees (Finz, 2004). However, when the Maxwell's created Power Bar, they included high fructose corn syrup as a principal ingredient. High fructose corn syrup is nothing more than a slow-acting poison that might have played a role in the death of Maxwell.

Check the ingredients on everything you eat and pray the labeling is accurate. Otherwise, be smart and eat raw fruits and vegetables. And if you want a quick pick-me-up, this would be a perfect time to rethink that health drink, power bar, or vitamin supplement pill. They shouldn't look so good anymore!

Chapter 19

The Perils of Physical Fitness

There is no question that physiological wellness at the cellular level is far superior to physical fitness. We've already discussed the fates of those who were supremely physically fit and still managed to die young or become afflicted with deadly diseases. Yes, it's good to be active, but that's not the same as working out at the local gym or buying fitness equipment that occupies half your home. Unless you're joining a gym because you're lonely or are a social animal that must show off your abs and pecs, a 20-minute stretch and indulgence in minimum-resistant exercises two or three times per week is just fine. All that hyper training at the gym might do your body far more harm than good and isn't a substitute for a healthy lifestyle that incorporates a raw fruits and vegetables diet.

Those Oh-So-Smart Trainers

Let's start with the personal or not-so-personal trainers who allegedly have your best interests and physical fitness at heart. Do they really? According to Certified Strength and Conditioning Specialist and Coach Molly Galbraith, "You may have been subject to slick marketing tactics or you may have been wooed by a Trainer with a great six-pack or a cute smile" (2014). Add to that the "wooing" they do to get you signed up and hooked on a fitness program.

As Ashwin Rodrigues humorously noted, "First of all, let me say if you are sensitive about your physical appearance, you should meet a personal trainer. They will say very nice things about you, because if they call you a fat idiot you may not return" (2014). I've incorporated parts of Ashwin's story here (with attribution) not just because it's hilarious, but because it truly describes, with no holds barred, the reality of gym fitness programs. That man worked out for twenty minutes before his "trainer," who knew nothing about nutrition, discussed his diet—questions about daily calorie intake and a recommendation that Ashwin eat "chicken, lots of vegetables, avocados, and other expletives, and take a multivitamin to be 'golden'" (the gym was partners with a supplement company that makes multivitamins and protein supplements) (Rodrigues, 2014). His trainer, by the way, limped due to an unrepaired ACL tear, which, to Ashwin, was like "seeing your mechanic driving away and one of his wheels fall off . . . your dentist only having two teeth . . . your librarian being illiterate" (Rodrigues, 2014).

Teacher Man (yes, that's his pen name) on YoungAndThrifty.com, says you don't need a personal trainer, and he doesn't understand why, at a time when the internet is all the rage and there are thousands of fitness magazines, people pay absurd amounts of money to have another person tell them how to do sit-ups and how many to do (Teacher, 2014). He goes on to state that personal trainers increase profits and engage in the "classic upsell that many gyms demand their personal trainers try to pursue" (Teacher, 2014).

Many gyms and companies give large commissions to trainers who get clients to purchase overly expensive supplements and a myriad of other high-cost products that are unnecessary and do you no good. Fitness is not wellness, and wellness doesn't come in the form of an exercise routine or a bottle of pills. It comes from eating healthy, which means a raw fruits and vegetables diet. Just don't tell that to your personal trainer. He/She won't agree with you, even though you're right.

Nasty Germs and Viruses

While it may come as a total surprise, gyms that promise fitness and health are actually breeding grounds for a smorgasbord of germs and viruses. Obviously, public places are a wellspring of those nasty contagions, but a gym is no different. According to the *Prospective study of bacterial and viral contamination of exercise equipment*, researchers found that 63 percent of gym equipment was infested with rhinoviruses (the cause of the common cold), cleaning and use of disinfectants didn't get rid of all the germs, and machines that were used by a number of people—one right after the other—might be the most difficult to keep totally clean (2006). The reason is that cold and flu germs and viruses have a longer lifespan on hard surfaces compared to rugs and other fabrics—up to 48 hours (Schwecherl, 2011).

Add to this the incidence of open wounds that come in contact with sweat, which makes athletes more vulnerable to skin infections, and that the most common "fitness bug" is staph bacterium MRSA, a significant cause of a serious skin infection (Schwecherl, 2011). While there was no proof that the staph bug came from machines, and likely came from body contact, it is recommended that embracing folks you don't know at the gym comes to a grinding halt (Schwecherl, 2011).

It gets worse. Gyms are breeding grounds for norovirus, which causes abdominal pain, vomiting, and diarrhea, and can live for one month on the surface of exercise machines (Reyes, 2012). Further, fungi that cause foot infections multiply exponentially in gym showers, while microbes like the antibiotic resistant MRSA bacterium (mentioned above) lies in wait in locker rooms (Reyes, 2012). Amesh Adjalia, a clinical assistant professor and a board-certified physician at the University Of Pittsburgh Medical Center who specializes in infectious diseases, believes that respiratory tract infections are the most common threat from gyms (Wooldridge, 2012).

A 2012 report from British researchers found that "communal fitness centers are basically like giant petri dishes," and almost 75 percent of those who go to gyms have seen poor hygiene take place all around them while they were working out—50 percent have shared water bottles and towels from time to time (Jio, 2012). Worse yet, the report indicated that "18 percent of people surveyed said they have no problem going to the gym with active colds, cough, and runny noses; and 16 percent said they don't wash their gym clothes between workouts, nor do they wear socks (Jio, 2012). A *Natural News* investigation revealed that fitness centers are warehouses of a profusion of dangerous germs that promote serious health risks including the common cold, diarrhea, and "even hepatitis A" (Wilson, 2014).

Natural News examined and revealed the 10 items that were the most germ infested, stating that they can survive on equipment for three days, even when sanitized twice a day (Wilson, 2014). Cardio equipment was home to germs like E. coli, fungi, yeast, and Staphylococcus aureus, "the prime cause of fatal hospital-acquired infections because of its high resistance to most antibiotics treatments" (Wilson, 2014). If you happen to get infected with the deadly E. coli, symptoms would include "severe stomach cramps, vomiting, and, in extreme cases, even kidney failure" (Wilson, 2014).

Swimming pools are another danger spot at gyms that have them. While the water is heavily chlorinated to kill or reduce bacteria, the water can contain cryptosporidium, a chlorine-resistant, microscopic parasite that causes diarrhea (Wilson, 2014). TV and radio devices are home to several dangerous bacteria. Locker rooms and showers harbor strep and staph bugs, and "fecal and other outdoor debris can be tracked in on shoes, causing warts, ringworm, athlete's foot, the flu, and even hepatitis A" (Wilson, 2014).

So why is there so little being done to protect fitness fanatics from the dangers of inappropriate fitness training and the diseases found at gyms? Follow the money. As early as 2005, ABC News reported on germ infestation at health clubs (Cuomo, 2006). According to microbiologist Dr. Philip Tierno, who aided in the investigation, the significant number of people, skin that's exposed, and the amount of sweat found at gyms create a perfect environment for spreading germs and infections (Cuomo, 2006). The undercover investigation included ABC News staffers taking swabs from almost every piece of gym equipment they used. Samples were then brought to Dr. Tierno's lab at New York University Hospital where he identified staph "aureus, sarcinia, candida specie, staphylococcus epi, diptheroids, klebsiella, enterobacter and E.coli" (Cuomo, 2006).

A Little Fitness Reality & Humor

You don't need to join a gym to increase your muscle strength in order to bench press 300 pounds or improve your ability to jog 15 miles. If you need to move a refrigerator or another very heavy object, ask for help or use a cart. If you need to go a distance in a hurry, ride your bike and peddle your way there, or get in your car and drive that distance. There is no reason to selfishly take time away every day from those you care about to jog or lift weights for hours. An individual's physical fitness goals should be practical and attained through physical wellness.

Life Lesson—Two Letters from Dr. S. R.

Dr. S. wrote to me twice. The first time was in 2003 after enduring back surgery and subsequent complications that required a five-week hospital stay. During our physical therapy sessions, I discussed body mechanics as well as responsible eating habits. He wrote, "I cannot begin to tell you how valuable your instructions on back care and diet have [been] to me. I have been able to lose over 25 pounds and have lowered my cholesterol over 95 points. Your passion and conviction for your back care and health prevention program are a true inspiration."

Two years later, when my classes at the hospital were discontinued ostensibly due to budget cuts, he wrote to the then CEO recommending they be reinstated. He wrote, in part, "Mr. Igani made a huge difference in my care. During my hospital stay, he went well beyond what would have been required of him as a hospital employee. Most importantly, he instructed me in nutrition and helped me change my lifestyle, both of which I found instrumental in my back care." It took a great deal of courage for a medical professional of his stature to stand up to the ruling powers, but he did because he knew I had shared with him a way to journey to wellness and the many productive years he had ahead of him.

The Whole Truth

Let's look at a few reasons we should strive to achieve physical wellness that don't require hours of exercise or jogging. Some will seem funny until reality takes over. It's good to be physically well so you can run out of a burning building or up a flight of stairs without experiencing shortness of breath or having a heart attack if the elevator is broken. It's good to be able to park far away from the entrance to a store so you can walk there instead of sitting in your car forever waiting for a spot to open up by the front door. It's really great to be able to park illegally or double park, run into your destination, get the errand done quickly, and get back to your car before the parking officer or meter maid gets there to right you a ticket.

Physical fitness as a subset of true wellness will allow you to outrun a tsunami and get to higher ground before you're washed away by a 20-foot wave. That same ability will serve you well if you're hiking or camping in the woods and you need to flee from a hungry bear. and if you are with people who are dishonest in their trades, you definitely want to outrun them to buy you more time to get to safety.

Some may call it selfish and uncaring, but I call it survival of "the wellest!" On that same note, you might want to outrun anyone chasing you if necessary, without experiencing shortness of breath. Finally, think about running a 100-meter dash and smoking your opponents who happen to be 10-20 years your junior. That's an example of a wellness moment that would uplift the spirits of even the most miserable person on the planet.

Well, I have some breaking news for all of you. I can do all of the above at age 53 and credit it to the food I consume daily. I am no superman, but I consume super foods that yield super performance! So what's a body to do? Eat healthy raw fruits and vegetables to achieve wellness. The best exercise is walking. You don't have to become obsessed with lifting weights, doing sit-ups, push-ups, or other stressful exercises to be healthy. What you need is a simple 20-minute stretch and indulgence in minimum-resistant exercises two or three times per week, as I noted at the start of this chapter. A couple of other exercises to improve your muscular and cardiovascular systems other than brisk walking are biking and swimming, if you can find a pool clean enough in which to swim. It's time to journey to wellness and leave fitness to those who don't understand the difference.

Chapter 20

"Trish's Story"

I started working with a middle-aged woman I will call Trish (to protect her privacy) in December 2006. She had a myriad of health problems when she first started her journey to wellness, all of which were leading her to a much shortened lifespan.

At age 24, Trish weighed 135 pounds and was extremely attractive. By age 52, she weighed 400 pounds and was in horrible physical condition. She was morbidly obese, in chronic pain, and horribly depressed. Trish was a physical and emotional time bomb who was totally dependent on pharmaceutical concoctions—both prescription and over-the-counter.

Her physical problems included shortness of breath, which was exacerbated by walking; use of oxygen at night and as needed; a CPAP machine (continuous positive air pressure) at night for seven years due to sleep apnea; asthma; fatigue after a 15-minute shower (which led to poor hygiene) or when walking short distances; narcolepsy (falling asleep frequently during the day); and chronic phlegm production, especially in the mornings. Those were just the breathing issues suffered by this woman who should have been out working and totally enjoying life.

Additional syndromes and illnesses included bladder leakage, severe pain in the weight-bearing joints when standing for over five minutes, chronic low back pain and pain in both heels when walking (plantar fasciitis), swelling in both feet (a strong indication of possible congestive heart failure), numbness and pain in both upper legs for the past two years, and depression and anxiety. There's more, if more is possible in one human being.

Trish also endured gastric esophageal reflux disease (GERD) and chronic constipation (since the age of five, lasting four to five days at a time), high blood pressure (140/80 while on two different blood pressure medicines), bruised easily due to taking Plavix (blood thinner), border-line diabetes (average blood glucose level was 70—164), three to four episodes of sudden weakness everyday due to blood sugar swings, frequent numbness episodes in hands and arms while driving and difficulty finding a comfortable chair in which to sit. Life was no fun for Trish because she was too busy dealing with all of her illnesses, syndromes, and conditions. Her prescription and non-prescription drugs included 39 doses of 26 chemical compounds, many taken more than once a day, and three medications taken as needed. The chart shows the medication, dosages, diagnosis, amount taken daily, and monthly and annual cost to the state:

Medication	*Dosage*	*Diagnosis*	*Frequency*	*Cost/Mo.*
Albuterol Inhaler		Asthma	as needed	25.79
Budesonide	0.4mg	Asthma	2x/day	197.90
Duoneb	3ml	Asthma	3x/day	349.99
Nasacort Spray		Asthma	2x.day	78.69
Provigil	240mg	Narcolepsy	2x/day	194.49
Singulair	10mg	Allergies	1x/day	101.19
Spiriva Inhaler		Asthma	1x/day	161.99
Buspirone	15mg	Anxiety	1x/day	112.59
Darvocet	100mg	Pain	as needed	56.49
Detrol LA	2mg	Bladder leakage	2x/day	228.99
Fluoxetine	40mg	Depression	1x/day	144.19
Furosemide	80mg	Edema	1x/day	15.19
Gabapentin	600mg	Pain	3x/day	166.19
Ibuprofen	800mg	Pain	3x/day	25.39
Lyrica	75mg	Pain/Neuropathy	1x/day	72.59
Metolazone	5mg	Edema	1x/day	40.19
Potassium	10mg	Potassium	1x/day	21.89
Risperdal	5mg	Anxiety	1x/day	265.39
Wellbutrin	300mg	Depression	1x/day	142.49
Diltiazem	200mg	Blood Pressure	1x/day	50.59
Levothyroxine	25mg	Thyroid	1x/day	12.09
Lisinopril	20mg	Blood Pressure	2x/day	63.29
Nitrolingual	0.4mg	Chest Pain	as needed	130.99
Omeprazole	20mg	Indigestion	2x/day	45.00
Plavix	75mg	Blood Clots	1x/day	155.89
Pravachol	80mg	Cholesterol	1x/day	154.89

The total cost to the state for Trish's medications was $3,014.36 per month for a total of $36,172.32 per year. This woman had become a costly, taxpayer-supported, chemical cocktail because of poor lifestyle and dietary choices. From the time she was 24 until she was 52, she had gained 252 useless, dangerous, and unhealthy pounds that added sickness upon sickness and a medicine cabinet filled with drugs that did nothing to change her conditions.

I was not her doctor, nor did I pretend to take on such a role. Working in concert with her doctors, I was a good friend who believed Trish could be healthier, happier, and a lot slimmer than she was when we started our "project" together. The Plan of Action for Trish focused on restoring proper enzyme functions, cell nourishment, and waste elimination. She had to cut out all supplements and eliminate the need for constipation remedies. Our goal was to get rid of her edema, chronic joint pains, normalize her blood pressure, eliminate her depression and anxiety, normalize her sleep and breathing patterns, improve shortness of breath, and increase her energy level.

Day 1

I was able to convince Trish to start changing her food consumption by eating 95 percent raw fruits, vegetables, and nuts. I also convinced her that almost all of the medications she was taking were the result of her poor eating habits. At that point I warned her that she faced serious risks and side effects from all those medications, but by improving her nutritional lifestyle she would also be able to decrease her need for almost all of the medications she was taking—an end to her dependency on pharmaceuticals. While Trish lamented that she had tried several different diets and remedies for years with no success, she admitted she was not happy with her physical condition and agreed to take my advice. After all, it didn't cost her anything since my advice was free. Again, it was the advice of a caring friend that was accepted by her doctors - they were in on the plan to save Trish's life.

Day 8

Trish noticed some major changes and improvements to her health that enabled her to reduce and eliminate some of her medications. Those decisions were made independently by Trish, herself. She related that phlegm production was no longer present, which allowed her to eliminate the use of Singulair, her allergy medication. She had less joint pain, which allowed her to eliminate Ibuprofen three times per day, Lyrica once a day, and Darvocet as needed. Her sleep quality improved helping reduce her narcolepsy. This led to a reduction in her use of Provigil from twice each day to once each day.

She also reported on Day Eight that she was no longer suffering from pitting edema in her ankles, which allowed her to eliminate her daily doses of Furosemide, Metolazone, and Potassium. Her breathing improved leading to the elimination of Albuterol, one of her "as needed" medications, and daily doses of Budesonide and Duoneb. What was amazing was her loss of food cravings and hunger and her increased energy level.

While Trish's bowel movements were still not regular and she did still suffer with periods of constipation, the consistency of her stools improved from painfully hard to soft. She also reported that she was urinating frequently, but not as often as she did when taking her diuretics. This explained the absence of the edema in the ankles. She was, however, concerned with the dark color of her urine, which led her to believe she might be dehydrated. I assured her that it's impossible to become dehydrated considering the amounts and types of fruits and vegetables that she was eating every day. I did explain that one of her medications may be responsible for the dark color of her urine. The good news was that she was able to legitimately eliminate the need for 16 dosages of medication in just one week on a plantarian diet. I suggested she continue as planned—eating more raw fruits and vegetables—to further reduce her constipation.

Day 12

Trish called to update me on her progress. She went to the doctor this day for her depression follow-up. She also stated she had been battling laryngitis and had not been able to talk for a few days, which led to her doctor prescribing the corticosteroid (anti-inflammatory) Methylprednisolone (4mg) and Avelox (400 mg), an antibiotic. There was, however, some great news. Her blood pressure had been reduced from 140/80 to 120/70, and she experienced less straining and more frequent bowel movements. She decided to eliminate Detrol LA, 2mg, 2x/day, and noticed that her urine color returned to normal. She also noticed that she has been able to begin to feel better faster with this episode of laryngitis than the previous ones.

In only 12 days on the plantarian diet, Trish made great strides towards improved health. At that point, I wanted to get a baseline weight on her, but her weight was not the most important factor, especially when I considered all the other improvements in such a short time. My only concern was that she would suffer from raw food fatigue and become discouraged, so I suggested she have one small portion of cooked food that I provided so she wouldn't feel deprived.

It was my belief that Trish had consumed enzyme-depleted foods for most of her life and, compounded with a dependency on artificial methods to improve bowel movements, suffered from sluggish peristalsis and chronic constipation. Our goal was to continue with the plan in order to establish normal metabolism, improved circulation, and softer consistency bowel movements at least two or three times per day. Trish did have one setback the next day. She opted to resume taking her Detrol LA after her bladder leakage symptoms returned. She did report continued progress in all other areas.

I knew that her weight was contributing to her bladder leakage. According to Obstetrician and Gynecologist Dr. May Wakamatsu, obesity is linked with incontinence (bladder leakage), especially for women because "the pelvic floor muscles must support excess abdominal fat as well as the pelvic organs, which can lead to stress incontinence (leaking when coughing or jumping)" (2010-2014). Obesity can put excess pressure on the bladder and block its blood supply (Wakamatsu, 2010-2014). Fat tissue may also contribute to an overactive bladder by changing the balance of chemical messengers between the nerve cells. Loss of weight can help improve incontinence (bladder leakage) without additional treatment (Wakamatsu, 2010-2014).

Day 16

Trish reported she experienced two large, soft bowel movements this day. The ring she's been unable to remove from her pinky finger for two years fell off on its own, and she can now bend her knees to 110 degrees instead of the meager 80 degrees she was able to flex two weeks ago. Over the past two years she lost the ability to curl her toes when sitting upright, but she reported she could finally do it with ease. Over the first two weeks of our plan, she had only taken two doses of Ibuprofen and had taken no Darvocet for pain. Her gas and bowel movements didn't have the unpleasant odor they did before she started the plantarian diet.

Her progress, which included improved flexion in both knees, her ring falling off the finger, and her ability to curl up the toes, were the direct result of reduced edema. According to the Mayo Clinic, edema is the swelling of specific areas of the body and is usually seen in the hands, arms, ankles, and legs, which could be a sign of specific underlying medical conditions (Godwin, 2013). While medical attention should be sought if edema continues for a long time, there are anti-oxidant rich fruits that can help those who either sit too long and/or eat too many salty foods (Godwin, 2013). Since Trish was on a rather strict plantarian diet, all of the progress she noted was indication that her body systems, especially her heart and kidneys, were operating more efficiently.

More frequent bowel movements and a lack of unpleasant odor were the result of her intestinal tract finally learning to empty waste in a timelier manner. This prevents prolonged time in the intestines where food waste continues to decay. Infrequent bowel movements, which were one of Trish's serious issues, indicated that fecal matter was moving through the intestines too slowly, providing more time for bacterial decomposition and absorption of water from the bowel (Loomis, 2014). Fecal matter then became dry and hard—the reason for Trish's chronic constipation—and the slow movement led to autointoxication as the bacterial and fungi/yeast were absorbed into the bloodstream, cleansed by the liver, sent to the kidneys, and finally eliminated (Loomis, 2014).

Day 17

There was more good news. Trish reported constantly having to pull her pants up because they were getting too big. Walking up her ramp became easier - she required only two stops to rest compared to three or four rests a week earlier. It was 7:00 p.m. and Trish had been out and about all day without needing any pain medication. Her chronic low back pain had almost disappeared. I instructed Trish to go out to eat once a week, which she said she did with her mother at Taco Bell—Nachos Belgrande with water at 4:00 p.m.

So, let's analyze the nutritional value of what Trish ate at Taco Bell. According to SparkPeople.com, one serving of Nachos Belgrande contains 760.0 calories, 42.0 g total fat, 8.0 g of saturated fat, no polyunsaturated fat or monounsaturated fat, 30.0 mg of cholesterol, 1,280.0 mg of sodium (not good at all), no potassium, 77.0 g of total carbohydrates, 12.0 g of dietary fiber, 5.0 g sugars, and 19.0 g of protein (2014). The sodium alone is a good reason for a headache, especially after two weeks on a plantarian diet.

There were absolutely no vital nutrients in Trish's Nachos Belgrande—no vitamin A, B-12, B-6, C, D, E, calcium, copper, folate, iron, magnesium, manganese, niacin, pantothenic acid, phosphorus, riboflavin, selenium, thiamin, or zinc (SparkPeople, 2014). Sounds like a waste of money to me and a great way to eat lots of nutritionally empty calories, a ton of sodium, and then down some Ibuprofen to clear up the headache that sets in within one day.

Day 18

Trish mentioned that she had a headache at the top of her head all day, which she attributed to a suspected spike in her blood pressure. However, when I checked her blood pressure, it was 125/70 with a pulse of 74 per minute. We both linked the possible cause of her lingering headache to the food she ate the day prior. It was possible that since her body had gone through a cleansing and detoxification process, high fats and high salty food could have shocked her system. I suggested that if the headache persisted through the evening she take an Ibuprofen. Trish reported taking one Ibuprofen at 8:00 p.m. Her headache improved but was not gone.

Day 19

Trish reported that she still had the headache and had to take another Ibuprofen, which was not doing the total trick. I suggested she take it easy and rest. She was also experiencing episodes of dizziness and weakness. There was no explanation for why she felt so bad except the meal she ate at Taco Bell. Clearly, the impurities in her meal and lack of nutrition contributed to her condition, which proved that processed, unhealthy foods were a large part of her physical problems. However, the combination of those foods and her antibiotics may have caused her setback as well.

Day 20

Trish called me to let me know that the antibiotics she was taking for her cold and laryngitis may have been be the source of her headache and weakness episodes. She discovered that some of the side effects include headache, dizziness, and stomach cramps. She was suffering from all three, but fortunately she had only two more days of antibiotics left. She did let me know that she was doing well in all other areas and would not take any Ibuprofen if she could tolerate the symptoms she was experiencing.

Day 21

Day 21 dawned with the end of Trish's headache, but she still had some weakness episodes. She also told me that she had only one slice of Stuffed Crust pizza from Pizza Hut and it had given her stomach cramps. I was not surprised. Fast, over-processed foods, as we've already discussed in prior chapters, do the body no favors. Trish was starting to get it. Her skin was getting looser all over her body. Her endurance improved when taking showers and she was able to reach and clean herself better. This is a terrible problem for morbidly obese individuals.

We know that obesity can contribute to illnesses such as hypertension, strokes, heart attacks, and diabetes (which can lead to skin lesions and infections), but it doesn't end there (Hill, 2013). Obesity can cause several different skin conditions including cellulitis and/or stretch marks, which also affect people who are not obese. However, other conditions are commonly found only among individuals who are obese, because the more overweight a person is, the greater the chance that issues of the circulatory system will affect the health of the skin and its function (Hill, 2013). In fact, a person's weight can produce pressure that breaks down the tissues of the skin (Hill, 2013).

Obesity can cause hygiene problems because of the amount of skin obese people must care for, and they may have trouble reaching some part of their bodies to perform good hygiene functions (Hill, 2013). When the folds of skin rub against each other, irritation occurs, which can lead to blisters and even chapping. An overload of moisture and perspiration doesn't help, nor does urine on the skin (which can lead to rashes) caused by poor hygiene and/or incontinence (Hill 2013).

Day 22

It is sometimes interesting to listen to patients who diagnose themselves. Then again, sometimes we know our bodies so well that we can diagnose ourselves. Trish mentioned that she had been constipated for about three days. She thought the Detrol LA was causing the constipation, but she had not been taking the full dosage. This led her to the decision to try to stop taking the Detrol LA to see if it was impeding proper bowel movements. To avoid problems, she decided to wear protective pads in case of continued bladder leakage. This was a very positive solution to a nasty problem.

Day 25

It had been three days since Trish took any Detrol LA and she had just finished the round of antibiotics for her cold. Since she had been so constipated for three days, she ate some prunes along with her daily fruits and vegetables. She was cleaned out like never before. She went from size 6X shirts to 4X very comfortably and her blood pressure went down to 114/57. Her joint pain was gone and she was able to reduce her blood pressure medication, Lisinopril (20mg), from 2x/day to 1x/day.

Day 27

Trish reported that she experienced a lot of stomach cramps. She hadn't been able to eat much food and occasionally snacked on a few cashews and small pieces of orange. She also reported having a couple of good, loose (no diarrhea) bowel movements that left her fatigued and totally cleaned out. She said she went to bed at 10:00 p.m. and didn't get up until 3:00 a.m., and took no medications for 24 hours. She felt well, except for her stomach, and her blood pressure was 125/85 with a pulse of 81—all without any blood pressure medicine. At that point, Trish decided to stop taking her blood pressure medicines, but I urged her to notify her physician prior to doing so, because it was far too soon to discontinue them. She agreed to continue taking Diltiazem (200mg) 1x/day and discontinue Lisinopril (20mg) 2x/day.

I saw more progress for Trish, who was able to sleep for five hours without needing her CPAP machine. She was also able to sleep without any feelings of suffocation. Her son noticed a dramatic change is her face, including a more defined bone structure. Trish's blood pressure was holding steady at 125/80 without any medications. I believed her stomach cramps were her body's response to the recent changes in her diet and her medications. I don't know why they didn't occur sooner, but she was back to feeling fine. I continued to monitor her blood pressure closely.

It's not uncommon for anyone to experience digestive distress when there's a major change in one's diet - such changes can actually shock the system, even if the change is a good one (Rose, 2013). For some people, vegetables, legumes, and other healthy foods come complete with several nutrients such as oligosaccharides, soluble fiber, and natural sugars, including fructose, which can sometimes create excess intestinal gas (Rose, 2013).

According to BodyEcology.com, vegetables are the most plentiful foods on earth and are also nature's most perfect foods—they are alkaline-forming and rich with vitamins and minerals the body needs to heal (2006). Raw vegetables are rich in enzymes, including those needed to help digestion. But after years of processed and junk foods, the digestive systems of many individuals are just too weak to digest all raw vegetables immediately, which means moderating the diet to add specific vegetables slowly as the digestive system is ready for them (BodyEcology, 2006).

Day 28

Day 28 started with Trish reporting severe joint pain in her knees and upper extremities that required one Darvocet. She also complained of nausea. I believed her joint pains were still associated with the flu she had two weeks ago. I encouraged her to stay the course and hopefully she would begin to feel better.

Day 30

Two days after experiencing her severe joint pain and nausea, Trish reported slight nausea, a decrease in the joint pain, and no sign or symptoms of blood pressure complications—it had been almost a week since she discontinued one of her blood pressure medications, Lisinopril 2x/day. Her blood pressure was 115/67 with only one blood pressure medicine. She had two small, soft bowel movements the day prior and one this day. She had reduced her prescription medications from 26 to eight; and on Saturday night, she slept seven hours without using her CPAP machine. She didn't use supplemental oxygen with the CPAP for five days. Trish also reduced her intake of Buspirone for anxiety and Gabapentin for nerve pain from 3x/day to 2x/day. These are remarkable changes and accomplishments for anyone, especially Trish.

Day 32

Things continued to improve. Trish reported feeling much better on Day 32 and said that the CPAP machine dried the mucus in her sinuses and throat. I suggested she make an appointment for another sleep study to determine whether the air pressure intensity could be reduced. The good news was that Trish hadn't taken Omeprazole for indigestion this day and she felt fine, but continued to take her nightly dose. She also did not drink any coffee for a week and suffered no signs of withdrawal from caffeine, and for the past week she's had one-two bowel movements per day. An important goal had been accomplished. She was now on her way to excellent health. I was very pleased and proud of her hard work.

Day 33

Trish stated she only took one medication for indigestion the day prior and was going to continue until she was totally weaned off of the medication. She also mentioned that she went to the store and walked around instead of using her wheelchair. That was a major milestone in Trish's journey to wellness.

One Month Update on Daily Medications

Medication	*Dosage*	*Diagnosis*	*Frequency*	*Cost/Month*
Buspirone	15mg	Anxiety	2x/day	112.59
Fluoxetine	40mg	Depression	1x/day	144.19
Gabapentin	600mg	Pain	2x/day	166.19
Levothyroxine	25mg	Thyroid	1x/day	12.09
Omeprazole	20 mg	Indigestion	1x/day	45.00
Spiriva Inhaler		Asthma	1x/day	161.99
Wellbutrin	300mg	Depression	1x/day	142.49

The total cost to the state for Trish's medications was 784.54 dollars per month for a total of 9,414.48 dollars per year. This was quite a change. Trish had only been following the lifestyle program for 33 days, which prior to she was taking a total of 29 medications with 39 doses per day. One month later she was able to reduce her medication dependency by 22 medications and 30 doses per day. I considered this a modern-day medical miracle.

Day 34

Trish had a follow-up sleep study done to see if her CPAP air pressure needed to be turned down. She was also weighed. While her weight was only one of several significant factors regarding her health and the need for improvement, I was more interested at the time in getting a rough idea of her excess fluid loss. The last weight she remembered was 400 pounds just before we started her lifestyle program.

Day 36

This was another day of exciting news. Trish stated that she was able to take a shower at the hospital after her sleep study was completed. She was able to stand in the shower and wash her hair, dry her hair afterward, and put her clothes on—all while standing. She noted that one year ago following a sleep study, she couldn't stand to wash her hair due to fatigue. She was weighed at the hospital and was now at 370 pounds for a total excess fluid loss of 30 pounds.

Sleep center technicians who conducted the sleep study told Trish that she kept her mouth open a lot while sleeping, but didn't give her any additional information. They said they would inform the doctor of the results and he would determine if the pressure of the CPAP needed adjustment.

Day 38

Trish reported low back pain and took one Darvocet because she couldn't tolerate the pain any longer. She thought the weather had something to with her pain.

Day 40

Trish mentioned that her knees and low back were hurting, but not enough to warrant taking pain medication. She said since she hadn't taken any pain medications for over a month, she fell asleep for two hours after taking one Darvocet a couple of days prior. Trish also said she had no more problems with a leaky bladder and only noted minimum leakage when she strained or had an occasional cough. She was able to carry her garbage down the ramp and walk back up the ramp without any rest stops. She said she hadn't been able to do this for months.

Her goal, at the time, was to start eliminating her depression and anxiety medications. She planned to start weaning herself from Wellbutrin, 300 mg 1x/day, and started to take the medication every other day during the first week. In the following weeks, she took the medication once every two days and then completely stopped taking the medication within a month.

Day 43

Trish complained of some low back pain, but she stated she was doing very well in other areas. She was less dependent on the CPAP machine and predicted she wouldn't need it much longer. She reduced her Wellbutrin down once to every other day and reduced her Omeprazole for indigestion down to once every other night.

Day 47

Trish told me she had an episode of diarrhea and wanted to know what I thought she should do. I told her to hold off on oranges and just eat some raw nuts and an apple or a banana. She called me back a few hours later to let me know that her diarrhea had cleared up. She also informed me of the latest progress—her hands and arms don't get numb any longer while driving and the steering wheel could be lowered all the way down without touching her legs. She said that if she continued to make progress, she would start driving her pick-up truck, which is much smaller than her van. She had to adjust the rear view mirror down because her whole body was slower due to less mass in her buttocks.

She went shopping for groceries with her mother and was able to help her mother carry the groceries in the house without getting short of breath or tired. She stopped taking Wellbutrin after she tapered off for a week—another medication taken off the list. She reduced her Omeprazole (indigestion medication) to once every two days. These might not seem like milestones to most people, but for Trish they were signs of incredible progress toward a healthier life.

Day 50

Trish told me she has not taken her Omeprazole (indigestion medication) for three days and that she planned to discontinue it. She was not suffering from shortness of breath, which allowed her to stop using her Spiriva inhaler once a day for asthma. Trish also noted that her bowel movements increased from one or two per day to two to three per day. Remember that, since she was five years old, she would go up to five days without a bowel movement. Clearly, her body had learned to eliminate waste, which accounted for so many significant improvements in her health.

Day 52

I was leaving Fresh Market at 1:30 p.m. and recognized Mayor Ramsey (this was in 2007) walking into the store. I remembered that he had attempted to initiate a program to improve the health of Hamilton County residents. I asked him to look over Trish's health progress journal and give me a call if he though my program could be utilized to improve the health of folks living in Hamilton County while reducing their dependence on pharmaceuticals. He said he would look it over and give me a call.

Day 53

Trish was taking her Gabapentin 1x/day instead of 2x/day since Saturday for leg pain, and Buspirone for anxiety only once a day instead of twice a day without any problems. She was no longer suffering from numbness in the left upper leg area, but the right upper leg was still a problem.

Day 53

Daily Medication Update

Medication	Dosage	Diagnosis	Frequency	Cost/Month
Buspirone	15mg	Anxiety	once/day	37.49
Fluoxetine	40mg	Depression	once/day	144.19
Gabapentin	600mg	Pain	once/day	55.40
Levothyroxine	25mg	Thyroid	once/day	12.09

Trish was now taking four doses of medicines daily. The total cost to the state per month was $249.17 with an annual cost of $2,990.04. Recall that just 53 days prior, Trish's medicines cost the state $3,014.36 per month and $36,172.32 annually. Her improved health saved the state $2,765.19 per month and $33,182.28 annually. In just seven weeks on a plantarian diet, Trish reduced her drug dependency and intake from 29 medications and 39 daily doses to four medications and four daily doses. On Day 61 of her journey to wellness, Trish reported that she could wear an ankle bracelet and necklace for the first time in a few years. The absence of swelling enabled her to do that.

While such rapid changes may not occur for everyone, the likelihood is that most individuals will start to feel they are on the road to true wellness in a relatively short amount of time. It doesn't take long for the body to recognize and absorb the nutrients in raw fruits and vegetables, and it doesn't take long for the body to eliminate all the processed and junk foods that have been piling up for years or even decades. That's what was happening to Trish. As her diet changed to include raw fruits and vegetables almost exclusively, her body was absorbing more nutrients and processing those nutrients far more expediently. It's as if she were actually starving for decades and was finally eating foods that changed her body's entire chemical process. No longer was she starving, she was being well nourished. The list that follows shows all the conditions, syndromes, and illness that no longer plagued Trish after just 53 days on the plantarian diet.

Health problems that no longer existed or had been reduced:

1. Use of oxygen at night and as needed
2. Bladder leakage
3. Gastric esophageal reflux disease
4. High blood pressure, 140/80 with two different blood pressure medicines
5. Border-line diabetes (blood glucose level was between 74-96)
6. Swelling in both feet (strong indication of congestive heart failure)
7. 3-4 episodes of sudden weakness daily due to blood sugar swings

8. Chronic constipation for 45 years with no bowel movements for up to 4-5 days at a time
9. Bruised easily due to Plavix, a blood thinner.
10. Chronic phlegm production
11. Had difficulty with good hygiene
12. Extreme fatigue after a 15-minute shower
13. Narcolepsy (falling asleep frequently during the day)
14. Frequent numbness episodes in hands and arms while driving
15. Couldn't find a chair that was comfortable (more comfortable while driving)
16. Numbness and pain in both upper legs (reduced to left leg only)
17. Shortness of breath, exacerbated by walking (reduced)
18. CPAP at night for 7 years due to sleep apnea (decreased dependency)
19. Asthma (reduced)
20. Fatigued when walking short distances (reduced)
21. Severe pain in the weight bearing joints when standing over five minutes (reduced)
22. Chronic low back pain (reduced), pain in both heels still persists when walking
23. Depression and anxiety (reduced)

Life Lesson—Trish's Doctor

Trish's doctor wrote to me in April 2007, thanking me for providing Trish with nutritional suggestions and encouragement. I guess her doctor, with whom I worked on this massive "project," was happy with the continuous changes in his patient. He wrote, "I have been able to successfully eliminate many of her prescription medications. She seems to have increased energy and vitality, reduced depression and anxiety, improved circulation, sleep quality, and decreased joint pain. She has also lost 40 pounds in just two months and her recent blood profile demonstrates her improved lifestyle choices. I recommend your program to anyone who is in search of excellent health."

I know that was a mouthful or two, but I wasn't the one who did the hard work. It was Trish who made the choices and worked steadily to improve her own life. I started her on the journey and she chose to keep traveling. To this end, I can't thank Trish enough. She had the courage and conviction to know she had to make a change in her lifestyle and she took a chance. I don't know if she continued to stick with it. I lost touch with Trish when one of her close relatives passed away, sending her into a bout of depression as often happens when death hits that close to home. I can only pray that she learned all she needed to learn and did not regress. She had far too much going for her and lots of years left if she continued on the road she was on. I hope she didn't give up her journey to wellness.

Chapter 21

What Goes In Must Come Out

I know it's a messy subject, but it must be discussed. I've often witnessed doctors turn a blind eye to the subject of bowel movements. It's never addressed in depth, especially if the patient has one bowel movement at least every other day. Health professionals don't seem to be interested in or concerned with the real cause of constipation. Instead, they are ready to prescribe something for quick relief.

It's a shame that constipation is a subject suffering individuals are interested in but are too uncomfortable to discuss publically. However, the ability to empty our bowels is just as important a body function as heart beats, the breaths we take, and the foods we eat. The inability to eat on a regular basis is a strong indication of a sick body and so is the inability to eliminate waste regularly. Remember, what goes in must, eventually, come out—the waste our body doesn't need must be eliminated.

Since it's just as normal as any other body functions, let's discuss it and deal with it. The truth is: relying on anything other than plants to relieve constipation creates a host of illnesses such as heart disease, stroke, diabetes, and sluggish bowels. As noted in a previous chapter, the majority of Americans attempt to function on a daily basis with an average of 16 pounds of fecal matter in their intestines. Minimal (a daily bowel movement) to severe constipation (every other day bowel movement) can affect just about every function of the body, from thought processes to actual physical movements.

The odor and consistency of fecal matter are directly related to a person's food source and the length of time it spends in the bowels prior to its expulsion. Food must stay in the body long enough to release all potential nutrients and leave the body when the brain signals the colon to empty out—usually following consumption of the next meal. The strong, offensive odor and hard consistency of the bowel movement is a true indication of the body's struggle to digest indigestible substances and the overall fragile health of the individual.

The vagus nerve is also called the tenth cranial nerve. It starts in the brain, continues down to the stomach, and supplies parts of the body including the brain, heart, lungs and different organs in the digestive system (WiseGeek, 2003-2014). Damage to this nerve can cause significant medical problems such as "trouble talking or swallowing, hearing loss, or heart or digestive problems. Bladder issues leading to incontinence are often reported in patients with vagus nerve damage as well" (WiseGeek, 2003-2014). Continuous constipation is frequently a symptom of nerve damage in this area because of the way the stomach and intestines contract. A damaged vagus nerve can also increase the production of stomach acid (WiseGeek, 2003-2014).

Those who suffer from even periodic constipation know what it's like to sit on the toilet and strain to force fecal matter from their bodies. Unfortunately, when straining is involved in a bowel movement, the individual is actually holding his/her breath and "bearing down," known medically as "a Valsalva's maneuver, where one forcibly exhales against a closed glottis, a part of the airways involved in allowing air entry to the lungs" (Jaimison, 2013). This increases pressure on the stomach and helps push the stool from the colon, but it doesn't end there. It also affects the circulatory system because "holding one's breath while bearing down causes a temporary increase in pressure inside the chest, which reduces blood flow to the heart." The heart rate is then decreased, whereby the blood volume that should be pumped to the rest of the body decreases (Jaimison, 2013).

Until the stool is successfully passed out of the body, there are several changes in blood pressure and heart rate that usually don't harm those who have healthy cardiovascular systems. While the Valsalva maneuver is sometimes used diagnostically for people with heart problems or to fix abnormal heart rhythms or chest pain, doctors warn their heart patients not to strain while attempting to have a bowel movement (Jaimison, 2013).

A study of over 93,000 women who participated in the Women's Health Initiative revealed that "constipation is a risk factor for cardiovascular disease in postmenopausal women," and investigators from the National Heart, Lung, and Blood Institute in Bethesda, Maryland, noted that constipation was linked to "age, Hispanic and African American descent, diabetes, high cholesterol, family history of heart attacks, high blood pressure, obesity, smoking, depression, low physical activity levels, and low fiber intake" (Jaimison, 2013). Researchers now suspect that severe constipation may actually activate an inflammation that could speed up the onset of cardiovascular disease when the body's white blood cells release cytokines due to "abnormal or excessive bacterial proliferation from the gut, which could be related to constipation" (Jaimison, 2013).

According to the National Digestive Diseases Information Clearinghouse, people who have less than three bowel movements a week are likely suffering from constipation, something experienced by approximately four million other Americans (Carrera, n.d.). Stools that are irregular, hard, and dry generally happen because waste moves very slowly through the large intestine, which permits water to be removed from the stool (Carrera, n.d.). Adding healthy fiber from raw fruits and vegetables to the diet allows the stool to move through the colon faster because water drawn into the colon makes the fecal matter softer and far easier to pass (Carrera, n.d.).

The Global Institute for Alternative Medicine holds that the high fiber in several fruits and vegetables supports healthy colon function by binding to toxins in the colon and preventing them from being absorbed (Roizman, 2014). Fiber also cleanses the body because it binds to bile acids in the intestinal tract so the bile isn't reabsorbed. This signals the liver to produce more bile, "which clears excess cholesterol out of your bloodstream and provides an avenue for the liver to dispose of toxins it has recently collected" (Roizman, 2014). The Harvard School of Public Health recommends approximately 20 grams of fiber daily for women and 30 grams of fiber daily for men—with that fiber coming from whole fruits, not juice (Roizman, 2014).

Most of the food currently consumed in the United States includes meat, dairy, and processed foods, all of which slow down the intestines and aggravate the mucosal lining in the digestive tract. Excessive mucous in the throat, sinuses, mouth, and tongue are clear indications that there's a build-up of fecal matter lining the digestive tract (OhMyRaw, 2013). Residue from the poor breakdown of processed foods, meats, dairy foods, and fast foods stays in the body and harms health (OhMyRaw, 2013). In fact, build-up in the colon makes it difficult for the body to absorb nutrients properly from even healthy foods until the colon is cleansed of all the harmful foods that have been ingested.

Raw fruits and vegetables produce a minimal to moderate amount of gas due to the presence of live enzymes and other nutrients. The gas produced is not foul smelling simply because raw plants do not stay in the intestines long enough to decay. That means there's no need to take that gas-be-gone pill or use a potpourri arrangement in the bathroom unless you've consumed dead animal and/or processed food products.

Keep in mind that waste accumulation in the body creates a serious physiological stress at the cellular level, which leads to noticeable changes and symptoms such as headaches, fatigue, poor energy, abdominal cramps, and so on. Just imagine being stuck in a traffic jam or being a judge in a court room trying to listen to litigating plaintiffs and defendants. A driver or a judge victimized by the symptoms of constipation is already suffering from severe internal physiological stress, and additional external stress (a driver stuck in a traffic jam or a judge attempting to rule on a long and tedious case) can create a volatile situation. However, when all body systems work harmoniously and in concert with each other, a person can handle any external stressors much more effectively and calmly.

By the way, if you're suffering from chronic constipation, I can and will guarantee that you are also suffering from heart disease, cancer progression, and many other diseases. So, haul out those fresh fruits and vegetables and start munching. It will taste great, help in your journey to wellness, and no one will ever tell you you're a constipated fool.

Chapter 22

Shopping for Plantarian Foods

Most people know very little about how to shop for raw fruits and vegetables. Placed in appetizing settings in produce departments of both regular and organic food markets, most of us have no idea what we're buying and whether it's even the freshest produce we can find. Remember, that those produce departments, as previously noted, make up only 10 percent of all supermarkets. Add to that the contentious arguments on both side of the genetically engineered (GMO) and irradiated foods issues and most consumers want to throw their hands up in disgust. After all, when you want to buy a tomato, you don't want to have to wonder where it was grown, under what conditions it was grown, and whether it was born from seeds that God put on the planet or those created in a laboratory, and how it was handled before it reached the local supermarket.

People who are extremely serious about their plantatrian diets, who eat mainly whole plants and a very small percentage of cooked or processed plants, will likely shop for organic produce or grow their own because they are highly opposed to genetically modified and irradiated foods, all use of pesticides, and man-made agri-engineering to more of what they don't consider healthy foods.

Those on the opposite side don't care where the produce came from or how it was grown and "processed" as long as it's edible. In their defense, my own great health and the continued health improvement of my clients are the result of consuming mainly conventional raw fruits and vegetables, regardless of origin or methods of transportation to the supermarkets. I have never consumed any produce that is labeled organic because, based on my observation and experience, plants mature and are fruitful only when all the nutrients are present in the right balance. Otherwise plants would not reach full growth, wouldn't be fruitful with normal looking fruits, and wouldn't taste familiar. I also believe that the nutritional benefits of such produce in disease prevention far surpasse the harmful side effects of the insecticide to which they are exposed.

Since I've laid out the differences between good lifestyle choices and poor lifestyle choices and left the decision with you as to which to choose, the smartest thing I can do (at this point in the book) is to give you both sides of the arguments regarding genetically engineered and irradiated foods and let you, the ultimate consumer of those products, decide for yourself.

What is Genetic Engineering?

Genetic engineering takes place when a gene from another source is inserted into another plant to create a plant that's supposedly better than it was before it was modified. Corporations that genetically engineer plant foods such as corn and soy, own the patents on those GMO seeds. Farmers have to buy new seeds each year—they sign an agreement not to reuse seeds from harvested crops—and more chemicals to continue their operations (Brassard, 2013). Non-GMO seeds have no patent and are bought on the open market, traded freely, and even harvested routinely from last-year's crops.

The GMO Process

There are two routine types of genetic engineering of food crops that involve weed and pest control. Plants, such as soy, are genetically engineered to withstand pesticides and herbicides such as those used by farmers—kill the weeds without killing the soy seedlings (Decuypere, 2014). Creating GMO seeds makes the plants resistant to pesticides and herbicides and increases profit for the companies that own the patents on both the seeds and pesticides. Corn experiences a different type of genetic engineering whereby the plant's genetic structure is changed to contain an insecticide called Bt (Bacillus thuringiensis), which comes from bacteria in the soil and which is produced in the corn to kill an insect's stomach cells (Decuypere, 2014).

GMOs and Health Pros and Cons

From an environmental standpoint, scientists at Cornell University noted that pollen from GMO Bt corn might blow onto milkweed plants and kill insects needed for pollination and to balance the environment. It's also been documented that Bt corn may be speeding up the advancement of "superbugs" for which there are no cures, and which are resistant to common insecticides (Decuypere, 2014).

However, researchers at The University of California in San Diego claim that "a toxic bacterium can be added to crops to make them insect repellent, yet safe for human use" (Duvauchelle, 2014). This would also lead to the reduction of pesticide chemical use on plants, which would lower human and environmental exposure to pesticides (Duvauchelle, 2014). Further, Oklahoma State University reported that increased GMO crops and animals require lower amounts of chemicals, as well as time, tools, lower environmental pollution, lower greenhouse gas emissions and create less soil erosion (Duvauchelle, 2014).

However, researchers at Brown University found that foods containing GMOs can create important risks of allergies because the process combines and/or adds proteins that are not native to the original plant or animal (Duvauchelle, 2014). Such blending or additions can lead to new allergic reactions in human beings, especially if the protein that's blended or added to the plant is something to which you're already allergic. The reaction isn't to the food you're eating, it's to what has been added to that plant or animal's genetic makeup (Duvauchelle, 2014).

The non-profit Center for Food Safety holds that 90 percent of the foods we consume contain some form of GMOs, especially if they're made with soy, corn, or other genetically modified crops with altered DNA (Colbert, 2014). Those products wind up in most of the foods we eat, whether it's a slice of toast, pizza, or a salad, and only those on organic-only diets do not consume any GMO products. Conversely, there are claims that some GMOs are higher in protein, calcium and folate so they're really not harmful (Colbert, 2014).

The Global Politics of Food from AmericanRadioWorks.com claims that "there are no inherent differences between foods produced from genetically modified (GM) plants and those from non-GM crops" (AmericanRadioWorks, 2015). The truth is that all living things are composed of DNA which has four building blocks called nucleotides. The pro-GMO forces claim that moving one segment of DNA from one organism to another organism does not equate to adding something foreign to the recipient. Instead, the change in genetic composition encourages the modified one to produce a desirable trait (AmericanRadioWorks, 2015).

Additionally, the new organism must be tested for its safety, especially if it's made from a recognized allergen; and no one has "substantiated" even one human death or illness from eating genetically engineered foods (AmericanRadioWorks, 2015). Perhaps it's just too soon to tell whether that statement is true. Further, any studies done, particularly by proponents of GMO foods, would discourage the finding of a link between GMO food consumption and illness and/or death.

While the U.S. Food and Drug Administration (FDA) claims that GMO plants must meet the same safety requirements as conventionally grown and organic foods, GMO foods may also be responsible for an increase immune suppression, cause resistance to antibiotics, and lead to cancer (Colbert, 2014). The National Center for Health Statistics revealed that "food allergies in children under 18 years of age jumped from 3.4 percent in 1997 to 5.1 percent in 2009 to 2011" (Colbert, 2014). Notwithstanding some questions regarding the wisdom of consuming or not consuming GMO products, the U.S. government does not mandate labeling of GMO foods, though Vermont and Maine were the first states to pass legislation that requires such labeling on any foods made in whole or part using genetic engineering, and legislation is pending in 28 other states (Colbert, 2014).

I have discovered through my own experiments and observations that removing animal products, such as meat and dairy from the diet, eliminates allergic reactions or the symptoms. Removing the allergens via removal of such products from the diet leads to less taxation on the body which ultimately strengthens the body's immune system to fight the allergens effectively. The increase in food allergies among our children could also stem from the increased consumption of ready-to-eat or processed, indigestible food products and nutritional supplements by the children and expectant mothers.

Notwithstanding the benefits of removing indigestibles from the diet, the primary reason why such legislation is pending is the outcry from the informed public. The Institute for Responsible Technology (IRT) is a global giant that teaches consumers, the general public, and policy makers about GMO foods and crops, and investigates the impact GMO foods can have on health, the environment, agriculture and more (Walia, 2014). The Institute noted that doctors have been advised by The American Academy of Environmental Medicine (AAEM) to prescribe diets free of all GMOs for their patients because of documented damage to organs, disorders of the immune and gastrointestinal systems, rapid aging, and even infertility (2006-2014). We simply don't know the long-term consequences, if any, from consuming GMO foods. To this end, I have always recommended a diet free of processed foods, regardless of their origin or their ingredients.

Conventional Farming

Conventional agriculture is the most common farming practice in the U.S. and confines itself to removing trees, readying the soil for planting via tilling, putting irrigation systems in place, and then planting crops. Conventional agriculture uses insecticides and pesticides to prevent insect infestation and/or animals from eating crops (Webber, 2014). It includes such crops as corn, wheat, rice, bananas, soy beans, and tomatoes, but problems exist due to the use of chemical fertilizers and spraying of insecticides. Further, some believe that conventional farming is reducing/depleting the Earth's soil supply (Webber, 2014). Fields are generally not allowed to rest on the seventh year so they can be replenished.

On a positive note, federal regulations make it doubtful that conventional produce will harbor harmful levels of pesticides by the time consumers purchase them, and conventional farmers argue that the manure used in organic agriculture contains harmful bacteria such as E. coli that could pose more of a safety threat to consumers (Webber. 2014). According to the National Research Council, the traces of pesticides left on conventionally grown products are unlikely to cause an increased cancer risk. Also, if fruits and vegetables are properly washed, most of the chemicals can be removed (Webber, 2014). There is currently no research that supports a claim that organic produce is better or safer than conventional produce; and the USDA's seal that a product is organic only confirms that it was produced organically (Webber, 2014).

Organic Farming

Organic agricultural production is used to produce food and fiber. When the FDA published rules in 1997 delineating the meaning of "organic," consumer groups were furious because GMOs, irradiated foods, and other processed foods were included in the definition (Decuypere, 2014). The rules were changed and republished in 2000 with far more rigorous requirements. In order to be certified as organic, food companies cannot use "irradiation, conventional pesticides, sewage sludge, fertilizers, petroleum-based fertilizers, or genetic engineering" (Decuypere, 2014). Animal products and by-products must come from animals that have not been given antibiotics or growth hormones, including rBGH (Decuypere, 2014). Farms where food is grown must be inspected by the USDA and all companies that handle or process organic foods prior to distribution in markets or restaurants, must also be certified as meeting USDA organic standards (Decuypere, 2014).

The advantage of organic foods is the freedom from antibiotics and hormones, no creation of toxic runoff into lakes, ponds, and streams which protects the environment, and better soil in which to grow crops. Buying from local producers helps the growth of sustainable farming where you live while protecting you from the dangers of GMOs, pesticides and other harmful substances that Big Agriculture is putting in your foods.

The Organic Center at Washington State University researches differences between conventional and organic farming in order to produce evidence that organic is better (Whole Foods, 2015). After investigating hundreds of studies, "they identified 236 scientifically valid 'matched pairs' of organic and conventional foods, and found the organic foods were nutritionally superior in 67% of the cases, vs. 37% for conventional" (Whole Foods, 2014). Organic Center researchers also found that "when a strawberry plant gets to grow without persistent pesticides – it produces certain phytochemicals to help do its own pest control. And new studies are finding that those chemicals may enhance the nutritional profile of the plant" (Whole Foods, 2015). Another recent study, however, indicates there is little difference in the nutrient content of conventional produce compared to organic produce. Researchers at Stanford University appraised approximately 250 studies that compared the nutrients found in organic vs. traditional fruits and vegetables (as well as grains, poultry, meat, and eggs) and the health outcomes of eating those foods. They found there was very little difference in the nutrient content other than somewhat higher phosphorous levels in many organic foods (Watson, 2012).

Today, organic products are no longer sold in the hidden corners of supermarkets because more consumers are going organic to avoid foods laden with antibiotics, as well as genetically engineered and irradiated foods. Organic agriculture is also better for the environment because it uses crop rotation, mechanical soil tilling and hand weeding, better mulching, and safer methods to stop weed growth (Webber, 2014). Even the USDA has noted that organic food products lowers input costs for farmers and reduces their dependence on nonrenewable resources while "removing about 7000 pounds of carbon dioxide from the air and [preserving] an acre of farmland per year" (Webber, 2014).

According to Marissa Lippert, M.S., R.D., there are two main reasons for eating organic: fewer pesticides and higher nutrients (2015). Lippert contends that pesticides can be absorbed into vegetables and fruits, which was substantiated by the Environmental Working Group's (EWG) review of approximately 51,000 USDA and FDA "tests for pesticides on 44 popular produce items and identified the types of fruits and vegetables that were most likely to have higher trace amounts" (Lippert, 2015). Lippert cited information from the Environmental Working Group regarding which foods have the highest or lowest levels of pesticide problems:

Preferably Organic*—Most Commonly Contaminated: Apples, Celery, Strawberries, Peaches, Spinach, Nectarines, Grapes, Sweet Bell Peppers, Potatoes, Blueberries, Lettuce, and Kale/Collard Greens (Lippert, 2015).*

If Budget Allows, Buy Organic*—Green Beans, Summer Squash, Peppers, Cucumbers, Raspberries, Grapes (domestic), Plums, Oranges, Cauliflower, Tangerines, Bananas, Winter Squash, Cranberries (Lippert, 2015).*

It's Your Call/Least Commonly Contaminated*—Onions, Sweet Corn, Pineapples, Avocado, Asparagus, Sweet Peas, Mangoes, Eggplant, Cantaloupe, Kiwi, Cabbage, Watermelon, Sweet Potato, Grapefruit, Mushrooms (Lippert, 2015).*

With regard to nutrient content, a 2007 Newcastle University study conducted in the UK reported that "organic produce boasted up to 40 percent higher levels of some nutrients (including vitamin C, zinc and iron) than its conventional counterparts" (Lippert, 2015). Further, a 2003 study in the *Journal of Agricultural and Food Chemistry* noted that "organically grown berries and corn contained 58 percent more polyphenols—antioxidants that help prevent cardiovascular disease—and up to 52 percent higher levels of vitamin C than those conventionally grown" (Lippert, 2015).

The study's lead author, Alyson Mitchell, Ph.D., an associate professor of food science and technology at the University of California, Davis, holds that higher nutrient content can be explained by the fertility of the soil and the plant's growth process. "With organic methods, the nitrogen present in composted soil is released slowly and therefore plants grow at a normal rate, with their nutrients in balance. Vegetables fertilized with conventional fertilizers grow very rapidly and allocate less energy to develop nutrients" (Lippert, 2015). In fact, buying local produce from local farmers means higher nutrient value because of its freshness and minimal travel time, regardless of its conventional or organic origin.

A Note on Radiated and Irradiated Foods

In 1986, the move to subject most of our foods to nuclear irradiation was given the okay by the U.S. Food and Drug Administration (FDA) which made it legal to irradiate vegetables, fruits, and spices (Colby, 2014). In 1990, the FDA permitted the same irradiation for poultry, in 1997, the irradiation process was extended to beef, lamb, pork, and horse meat, and finally to "fresh shell eggs" in 2000 (Colby, 2014). There is now an FDA move to irradiate all shellfish, meat that isn't refrigerated, alfalfa and sprouts from seeds, which means that 90 percent of what the average American eats will be irradiated (Colby, 2014).

What does this mean for the consuming public? What irradiation is doing is masking the real causes of food contamination such as "inhumane factory farming practices, corporate food monopolies with a single-minded fixation on profit, dramatic cutbacks in federal food safety inspectors, dangerous processing and slaughtering facilities, and a citizenry increasingly disconnected from local, sustainable food sources" (Colby, 2014).

Now that you're armed with information, both pro and con, regarding how plant foods are grown and brought to market, it's up to you to decide what you will eat so you can journey to wellness. Don't be afraid to ask the manager of your local produce department about the products on the shelves. Most of all, buy the foods that will make your plantarian diet something you enjoy; and do your homework. New information and technologies are always at the forefront of the news, but it's up to you to sort out fact from fiction.

Keep in mind that you don't have to worry about any harmful side effects from genetically modified organisms, pesticides, or irradiated foods if you smoke, are involved in the daily minimal-to-moderate consumption of alcohol, animal products, nutritional supplements, and processed foods, or dine out at a fast food restaurant at least once or twice per week. Conventional or organic is irrelevant because those irresponsible behaviors are causing just as much havoc if not worse on your entire vascular system, which is the origin of great health or disease, and study after study documents the strong link between animal food source consumption and disease.

A strong message to keep in mind from the bottom of my disease-free heart to all of loyal animal lovers of the world: it shouldn't be difficult to love all types of animals and none should ever find themselves on our dinner plate.

Postscript

I came to America as a teenager, longing for freedom and opportunity. While my early years here were sometimes trying and frustrating, I studied, attended school, earned a college degree, worked hard, and became part of the physical therapy field as a physical therapist assistant. However, over the past almost 40 years since my arrival in this country, I've watched as many of our God-given freedoms have been slowly eliminated or buried under volumes of regulations.

This nation allows its citizens a great deal of personal choice, especially on personal issues - but we are not necessarily a free people. Freedom to choose isn't the same as making personal choices, especially when those choices impact the lives of others. When personal lifestyle choices affect my freedom of movement, association with others, or my bank balance, I am no longer free. While some want no government regulations, our irresponsible behaviors are leading us to a day when the government will control us completely—from what we think to what we eat. Better to stop that encroachment by government now before it's too late. That means we must make better lifestyle choices.

I believe our elderly citizens deserve outstanding medical care and the freedom to choose a healthy diet that will lead them to the wellness that's been denied to them so long by the government-medical-pharmaceutical-insurance complex. I believe our children should be free to eat healthy foods that taste good, are nutritious, produce wellness, and cost less than a Big Mac. Mostly, I believe all Americans must be free of government-sanctioned, corporate brainwashing and regulations regarding our food choices.

The lies simply must stop. We must stop believing that our children have to eat specific foods to be socially accepted. We must stop pandering to the lowest levels of foods that are neither nutritious nor digestible, and start insisting that corporate food growers and manufacturers stop manipulating our food sources and contaminating them with harmful products.

I have worked tirelessly to write a book that would educate you and inspire you to achieve true wellness and freedom from archaic, non-productive, and harmful methods of eating. I hope I have communicated the information in such a way that going food shopping is no longer a chore or a hit-and-miss, just fill-the-shopping-cart experience. My prayer is that from this day forward, shopping for food will become something joyous and you choose the best foods with the highest nutrition—a smorgasbord of raw fruits and vegetables—that will help your bodies heal, maintain optimal wellness, and set you free from diets, scams, and phony scientific claims that amount to nothing but empty promises bordering on fraud. May you enjoy and celebrate your journey to wellness. Anything less is only half a life.

REFERENCES BY CHAPTER

Chapter 2: Wellness Accountability

Alcohol and Your Health. (2014). *HealthCheckSystems.* Retrieved from http://www.healthchecksystems.com/alcohol.htm

Cass, H., M.D. (2014). *Nutritional Approaches to Mental Health. GlobalHealingCenter.* Retrieved from http://www.globalhealingcenter.com/nutrition/nutritional-approaches-to-mental-health

Clower, W., M.D. (2014). *Don't Blame Big Food For Our Health Problems, Just Stop Buying Crap. MindBodyGreen.* Retrieved from http://www.mindbodygreen.com/0-15399/ dont-blame-big-food-for-our-health-problems-just-stop-buying-crap.html

Denton, C., L.N. (2013). *How Does Food Impact Health? Taking Charge of Your Health & Wellbeing.* University of Minnesota. Retrieved from http://www.takingcharge.csh.umn.edu/explore-healing-practices/food-medicine/how-does-food-impact-health

F. E., Dr. (2014). *Nutritional Approaches to Mental Health. Global Healing Center.* Retrieved from http://www.globalhealingcenter.com/natural-health/nutritional-approaches-to-mental-health/

Fleck, A. (n.d.). *Children With Poor Nutrition. Healthy Eating.* SFGate. Retrieved from http://healthyeating.sfgate.com/children-poor-nutrition-6555.html

Gunnars, K. (2012-2014). *11 Graphs That Show Everything That is Wrong With The Modern Diet.* Authority Nutrition. An Evidence-Based Approach. Retrieved from http://authoritynutrition.com/11-graphs-that-show-what-is-wrong-with-modern-diet/

Johnson RJ, et al. (2007). *Potential role of sugar (fructose) in the epidemic of hypertension, obesity and the metabolic syndrome, diabetes, kidney disease, and cardiovascular disease.* The American Journal of Clinical Nutrition. Retrieved from http://ajcn.nutrition.org/content/86/4/899.full.pdf

Plesman, J. (2011). *Drug Addiction is a Nutritional Disorder.* Hypoglycemic Health Association. Retrieved from http://www.hypoglycemia.asn.au/2011/drug-addiction-is-a-nutritional-disorder/

Smith, M. (2012). *Alcohol can lead to malnutrition.* Michigan State University Extension. Retrieved from http://msue.anr.msu.edu/news/alcohol_can_lead_to_malnutrition

Chapter 3: Body Chemistry

Bridgeford, R. (2012). *12 Reasons to Avoid Acids and Stay Alkaline. Alkaline* Diet Blog. Retrieved from http://www.energiseforlife.com/wordpress/2006/07/25/12-reasons-to-avoid-acids-and-stay-alkaline/

Haas, E., M.D. (2005-2014). *Elson Haas on Detox and Cleansing. Pure Inside and Out.* Retrieved from http://www.pureinsideout.com/elson-haas-detox.html

Chapter 4: Poor Lifestyle Choices and Body Chemistry

Banks, W.A. (2008). *The blood-brain barrier as a cause of obesity.* PubMed.gov. US National Library of Medicine. National Institutes of Health. Retrieved from http://www.ncbi.nlm.nih.gov/pubmed/18673202.

Dwyre B. (2013). *25 years ago: Pete Maravich's tragic trip to Pasadena.* Los Angeles Times. Retrieved from http://articles.latimes.com/2013/jan/05/sports/la-sp-dwyre-20130105.

Goldaper, S. (1985). *John B. Kelly Jr. Dead At 57; Olympic Committee Leader.* The New York Times. Retrieved from http://www.nytimes.com/1985/03/04/sports/john-b-kelly-jr-dead-at-57-olympic-committee-leader.html.

Gross, J. (1984). *James F. Fixx Dies Jogging; Author On Running Was 52.* The New York Times. Retrieved from http://www.nytimes.com/1984/07/22/obituaries/james-f-fixx-dies-jogging-author-on-running-was-52.html.

Hughes, R. (2011). *Glycemic Index: The Sweet Side of Life. GIAMTV. Health and Longevity.* Retrieved from http://www.gaiamtv.com/article/glycemic-index-sweet-side-life.

Story, C. (2012). *Heart Disease in Children.* Healthline. Retrieved from http://www.healthline.com/health/heart-disease/in-children.

Teasing and Bullying of Obese and Overweight Children: How Parents Can Help. (2013). American Academy of Pediatrics. Retrieved from http://www.healthychildren.org/ English/health issues/conditions/obesity/Pages/Teasing-and-Bullying.aspx.

Chapter 5: Through the Age Groups

Adams, M. (2010). *If mainstream medicine really works, why are Americans so unhealthy?* Natural News. Retrieved from http://www.naturalnews.com/028561_mainstream_ medicine_health_care.html#.

Americans Are Concerned about Poor Eating Habits. (2014). Barna Group. Retrieved from https://www.barna.org/barna-update/culture/677-americans-are-concerned-about-poor-eating-habits#.VGVK6DTF8YE.

Child Health Safety. (2010). WordPress. Retrieved from http://childhealthsafety.files. wordpress.com/2009/02/vaccines-did-not-save-us-e28093-2-centuries-of-official-statistics.pdf.

Chronic Disease Statistics. (2011). The Center for Managing Chronic Disease. University of Michigan. Retrieved from http://cmcd.sph.umich.edu/statistics.html.

Health, United States, 2013, In Brief. (2013). Centers for Disease Control. Retrieved from http://www.cdc.gov/nchs/data/hus/hus13_InBrief.pdf.

Heart Disease Facts. (2014). Centers for Disease Control (citing National Center for Chronic Disease Prevention and Health Promotion, Division for Heart Disease and Stroke Prevention). Retrieved from http://www.cdc.gov/heartdisease/facts.htm.

Lende, D. (2012). *Why Does the United States Rank So Badly in Health?* Neuroanthropology. Retrieved from http://blogs.plos.org/neuroanthropology/2012/08/12/why-does-the-united-states-rank-so-badly-in-health/.

Mundorff, Dr. L. (2014). *Why Is The American Diet So Full Of Unhealthy Foods?* Natural Savvy. Retrieved from http://naturallysavvy.com/eat/why-do-americans-eat-so-poorly.

Thompson, D. (2013). *Americans Still Making Unhealthy Choices*: CDC. Health. U.S. News & World Report. Retrieved from http://health.usnews.com/health-news/news/articles/2013/05/21/americans-still-making-unhealthy-choices-cdc.

Chapter 6: Nutrient Myths and Fairy TalesS

Axe, Dr. (2014). *Stop Using Canola Oil Immediately!* Retrieved from http://draxe.com/canola-oil-gm/
Campbell, T. C. & Campbell II, T.M. (2006). The China Study. Benbella Books. Dallas. Texas

Chatsko, M. (2014). *Truth behind 5 misleading food labels.* USA Today. Retrieved from http://www.usatoday.com/story/money/personalfinance/ 2014/08/17/ the-truth-behind-five-misleading-food-labels/14135379/

Coleman, C. (2012). *Juicing can wreck your looks: Flaking skin, hair loss and rotting teeth.* Daily Mail. Retrieved from http://www.dailymail.co.uk/ femail/article-2168872/Juice-diet-Flaky-skin-hair-rotten-teeth-The-latest-dieting-fad-pretty-ugly-effects.html

Diabetes: Sounding The Alert On A Debilitating Disease. (2008). Centers for Disease Control. Retrieved from http://cdc.gov/Features/DiabetesAlert/

Gunners, K. (2014). *6 Ways "Heart-Healthy" Whole Wheat Can Destroy Your Health.* Authority Nutrition, Retrieved from http://authoritynutrition.com/6-ways-wheat-can-destroy-your-health/

High-Temperature Cooking & The World's Healthiest Foods. (2014). whfoods.org. Retrieved from http://www.whfoods.com/genpage.php? tname=george&dbid=122

Institute for Responsible Technology. (2006-2014). 10 Reasons to Avoid GMOs. Retrieved from http://www.responsibletechnology.org/10-Reasons-to-Avoid-GMOs

Isaacs, T. (2012). *A tragic and stunning case of scientific fraud in studies on red wine and resveratrol.* Natural News. Retrieved from http://www.naturalnews.com/035315_red_wine_resveratrol_scientific_fraud.html

Kam, K. (2014). *Cravings: Why They Strike, How to Curb Them.* WebMD. Retrieved from http://www.webmd.com/diet/features/cravings-why-they-strike-what-to-do

Kirkey, S. (2014). *Drinking milk not essential for humans despite belief it prevents osteoporosis, nutritionist says. Appetizer.* National Post. Retrieved from http://life.nationalpost.com/2014/01/23/ drinking-milk-not-essential-for-humans-despite-belief-it-prevents-osteoporosis-nutritionist-says/

McAfee, M. (2012). *The 15 Things That Milk Pasteurization Kills.* The Campaign for Real Milk. Retrieved from http://www.realmilk.com/commentary/15-things-that-milk-pasteurization-kills/

Med diet helps prevent diabetes. (2008). BBC News. Retrieved from http://news.bbc.co.uk/2/hi/health/7426326.stm

Myers, A., M.D. (2014). *The Dangers of Dairy.* Retrieved from http://www.amymyersmd.com/2013/04/12/the-dangers-of-dairy/

Offit, P. (2013). *The Vitamin Myth: Why We Think We Need Supplements. Health.* The Atlantic. Retrieved from http://www.theatlantic.com/health/archive/2013/07/ the-vitamin-myth-why-we-think-we-need-supplements/277947/

Parker-Pope, T. (2007). *The Problem with Chocolate.* New York Times. Retrieved from http://well.blogs.nytimes/com/2007/1/21/the-problem-with-chocolate

Richards, G. (2011). *Pregnancy Myths Busted! Babble.* Retrieved from http://www.babble.com/pregnancy/pregnancy-myths-busted/

Robin, S. (2014). *Health Benefits of Nuts: Raw vs. Roasted. Healthy Eating.* SF Gate. Demand Media. Retrieved from http://healthyeating.sfgate.com/ health-benefits-nuts-raw-vs-roasted-3920.html

Spencer, B. (2014). *Moderate drinking IS bad for your health: Just two glasses of wine a day can cause problems.* The Daily Mail. Retrieved from http://www.dailymail.co.uk/health/article-2688161/Moderate-drinking-IS-bad-health-Just-two-glasses-wine-day-cause-problems.html

Wang, S. (2011). *Is This the End of Popping Vitamins?* In The Lab. Health and Wellness. The Wall Street Journal. Retrieved from http://online.wsj.com/articles/SB10001424052970204644504576650980601014152

Chapter 7: The Tidal Wave of Nutrients

Alternatives For Stroke Prevention: Nutrition and Diet. (2014). Alternative-Health-Group .org. Retrieved from http://www.alternative-health-group.org/stroke.php

Bollacker, J. (2012). *Six Reasons to Eat More Cabbage.* Full Circle. Retrieved from http://www.fullcircle.com/goodfoodlife/2012/09/22/six-reasons-to-eat-more-cabbage/

Boulanger, A. (2013). *Health Benefits Of Blueberries: 5 Reasons To Eat More Blueberries.* Medical Daily. Retrieved from http://www.medicaldaily.com/health-benefits-blueberries-5-reasons-eat-more-blueberries-246727

Bruso, J. (2014). *What Are the Benefits of Eating Pineapple?* Livestrong. Retrieved from http://www.livestrong.com/article/412290-what-are-the-benefits-of-eating-pineapple/

Busch, S. (2014). *What Is Acerola Cherry?* Sun-Sentinel. Retrieved from http://www.livestrong.com/article/115854-acerola-cherry/

Campbell, T.C., PhD. (2013). *Animal vs. Plant Protein,* Center for Nutrition Studies. Retrieved from http://nutritionstudies.org/animal-vs-plant-protein/

Campbell, T.C., PhD & Campbell T. M., II (2006). *The China Study.* Benbella Books. Dallas, Texas.

Coffman, M.A. (n.d.). *What Are the Benefits of Eating Oranges?* Healthy Eating. SFGate. Retrieved from http://healthyeating.sfgate.com/benefits-eating-oranges-4445.html

Daniluk, J., R.H.N. (2014). *5 healthy reasons to eat more fresh strawberries.* Chatalaine. Retrieved from http://www.chatelaine.com/health/diet/five-health-reasons-to-eat-more-fresh-strawberries/

Davis, J.L. (2005-2014). *Cranberries: Year Round Superfood.* WebMD. Retrieved from http://www.webmd.com/food-recipes/features/cranberries-year-round-superfood

Elliot, S. (1998-2014). *Lovely Lycopene: 5 Hidden Health Benefits of Tomatoes.* HowStuffWorks. Retrieved fromhttp://recipes.howstuffworks.com/fresh-ideas/healthy-dinners/5-hidden-health-benefits-of-tomatoes.htm

Harvard Health Publications. (2007). *Vitamin D and your health: Breaking old rules, raising new hopes.* Harvard Medical School. Retrieved from http://www.health.harvard.edu/newsweek/vitamin-d-and-your-health.htm

Herrington, D. (2012). *9 Health Benefits of Broccoli.* Care2. Retrieved from http://www.care2.com/greenliving/love-it-or-hate-it-broccoli-is-good-for-you.html

Knutson, P. (2014). *Is Vegan Vitamin B12 REALLY Necessary?* Vegan Coach. Retrieved from http://www.vegancoach.com/vegan-vitamin-B12.html

Lewin, J. (2014). *The health benefits of... spinach.* BBC GoodFood. Retrieved from http://www.bbcgoodfood.com/howto/guide/ingredient-focus-spinach

Lewis, A. (2012). *Top 10 Health Benefits of Eating Kale.* MindBodyGreen. Retrieved from http://www.mindbodygreen.com/0-4408/Top-10-Health-Benefits-of-Eating-Kale.html

MNT (2014). *What are the health benefits of avocados?* MediLexicon International, Ltd. Retrieved from http://www.medicalnewstoday.com/articles/270406.php

MNT (2014). *What are the health benefits of papaya?* MediLexicon International, Ltd. Retrieved from http://www.medicalnewstoday.com/articles/275517.php

Nutrient Composition of Plant and Animal-Based Foods (per 500 calories of energy). (2014). TheVeganRoad. Retrieved from http://theveganroad.com/health-fitness/principles-of-plant-based-nutrition-principle-3/

Principles of Plant-Based Nutrition. (2014). The Vegan Road. Retrieved from http://theveganroad.com/health-fitness/principles-of-plant-based-nutrition-principle-3/

Road to a Healthy Heart. (n.d.). Chart 11.2: Nutrient Composition of Plant and Animal-Based Foods (Per 500 Calories of Energy). Retrieved from http://road2healthyheart.com/uploads/3/2/3/0/3230638/nutrition_chart.pdf

Rogers, J. (n.d.). *10 Powerful Health Benefits of Parsley.* Natural Alternative Remedy. Retrieved from http://www.naturalalternativeremedy.com/10-powerful-health-benefits-of-parsley/

Sarao, C. (2013). *Benefits of Raspberries.* Livestrong. Retrieved from http://www.livestrong.com/article/419257-benefits-of-raspberries/

Scutti, S. (2013). *Health Benefits Of Peaches: Calories And Other Nutritional Information.* Medical Daily. Retrieved from http://www.medicaldaily.com/health-benefits-peaches-calories-and-other-nutritional-information-246755

Swalin, R. (2014). *5 Things You Didn't Know About Watermelon.* ABC News.com. Retrieved from http://abcnews.go.com/Health/Wellness/things-didnt-watermelon/story?id=24420280

Szalay, J. (2014). *Bananas: Health Benefits, Risks & Nutrition Facts.* Live Science. Retrieved from http://www.livescience.com/45005-banana-nutrition-facts.html

The Joyful Elephant (n.d.). Why is a plant-based diet so advantageous? JoyfulElephant.com. Retrieved from http://www.joyfulelephant.com/plant-based-diet-advantages.html

Thompson, C. (2005-2014). *5 Fun Facts About Carrots.* WebMD. Retrieved from http://www.webmd.com/food-recipes/features/5-healthy-facts-about-carrots

Tuso, P.J., M.D. (2013). *Nutritional Update for Physicians: Plant-Based Diets,* Permanente Journal, US National Library of Medicine, National Institutes of Health. Retrieved from http://www.ncbi.nlm.nih.gov/pmc/articles/PMC3662288/

MNT (2014). *What are the health benefits of avocados?* MediLexicon International, Ltd. Retrieved from http://www.medicalnewstoday.com/articles/270406.php

Chapter 8: Medical Myths and Tall Tales

Adams, M. (2012). *What's really in vaccines? Proof of MSG, formaldehyde, aluminum and mercury.* Natural News. Retrieved from http://www.naturalnews.com/037653_vaccine_additives_thimerosal_formaldehyde.html#

Allen, A.C. (2014). *Countries spending the most on health care.* USA Today. Retrieved from http://www.usatoday.com/story/money/ business/2014/07/07/countries-spending-most-health-care/12282577/.

Alston, W.D. (2009). *Why Do People Get Flu Shots?* LewRockwell.com. Retrieved from http://www.unz.org/Pub/LewRockwell-2007oct-00032?View=Search

Bottled Water. (2008). Natural Resources Defense Council. Retrieved from http://www.nrdc.org/water/drinking/qbw.asp.

Desmon, S. (2008). *Smokers' genetic 'double whammy'.* The Baltimore Sun. Retrieved from http://articles.baltimoresun.com/2008-04-03/news/0804030076_1_smoking-causes-lung-developing-lung-lung-cancer

Empty Cradles / Q&A With Michael Lu: Fighting disparities in infant mortality. (2011). Milwaukee-Wisconsin Journal Sentinel. Retrieved from http://www.jsonline.com/news/health/120032294.html

Hering, B. (2005-2012). *Warn Men About Testicular Cancer Symptoms.* Volunteer Guide. Retrieved from http://www.volunteerguide.org/minutes/service-projects/testicular-cancer.

Lalumandier, J., DDS, MPH & Ayers, L.W., M.D. (2000). *Fluoride and Bacterial Content of Bottled Water vs Tap Water. American Medical Association.* Retrieved from http://courses.washington.edu/h2owaste/bottled_water.pdf.

MBD. (2013). *Scientists Finally Discover The Function of the Human Appendix.* Political Blindspot. Retrieved from http://politicalblindspot.com/scientists-finally-discover-the-function-of-the-human-appendix/.

More Flu Vaccine Aimed at Key Spreaders: Kids. (2008). USA Today. Retrieved from http://usatoday30.usatoday.com/news/health/2008-09-08-flu-vaccine_N.htm.

Nutrition and Colon Cancer. (2001-2014). Johns Hopkins Colon Cancer Center. Retrieved from http://www.hopkinscoloncancercenter.org/CMS/ CMS_Page.aspx?CurrentUDV=59&CMS_Page_ID=8345F49E-9814-467C-B7F3-A68FC4c6FE96.

USA's 4th Leading Cause of Death—Pharma's Drugs. (2012). Child Health Safety. Retrieved from https://childhealthsafety.wordpress.com /2012/06/25/4th-leading-us-cause-of-death-pharmas-drugs/.

Wazana, A., M.D. (2000). *Physicians and the Pharmaceutical Industry, Is a gift ever just a gift?* Journal of the American Medical Association. Retrieved from http://med.stanford.edu/coi/journal% 20articles/ Wazana_A-Is_A_Gift_Ever_Just_A_Gift.pdf.

Williams, D., Dr. (2014). *Q&A: Should You Have Your Appendix Removed?* Retrieved fromhttp://www.drdavidwilliams.com/should-you-have-appendix-removed/

Chapter 9: Do You Trust Your Doctor?

Buchan, W. (1784). *Domestic medicine, or, A treatise on the prevention and cure of diseases by regimen and simple medicines: with an appendix, containing a dispensatory for the use of private practitioners.* Philadelphia. Retrieved from http://www.nlm.nih.gov/exhibition/georgewashington /digitalgallery/detail-buchan-book.html

Campbell, E. G, Ph.D., Gruen, R. L., M.D., Ph.D., Mountford, J., M.D., Miller, L.G., M.D., Cleary, P.D. Cleary, Ph.D., and Blumenthal, D. M.D., M.P.P. (2007). *A National Survey of Physician–Industry Relationships.* Vol 356:1742-1750, Number 17. Retrieved from http://content.nejm.org/cgi/content/short/356/17/1742

Cicala, R., M.D. (2003). *Substance Abuse Among Physicians: What You Need to Know.* Hospital Physician, pp. 39-46. Retrieved from http://www.turner-white.com/pdf/hp_jul03_know.pdf

Day, J. (2014). *Why I Don't Trust Doctors.* Retrieved from http://chetday.com/donttrustdoctors.htm

Hippocratic Oath. (2014). Wikipedia. Retrieved from http://en.wikipedia.org/wiki/Hippocratic_Oath

Krupa, C. (2012). *15% of surgeons struggle with alcohol problems.* American Medical News. Retrieved from http://www.amednews.com/article/20120306/profession/303069998/8/

Lasagna, L. (1964). *Tufts University School of Medicine, cited in Hippocratic Oath.* (2010). Johns Hopkins Sheridan Libraries. Retrieved from http://guides.library.jhu.edu/content.php?pid=23699&sid=190964

Parikh, R. (2011). *Why does your doctor hate alternative medicine?* Salon.com. Retrieved from http://www.salon.com/2011/05/02/alternative_medicine_and_doctors_oz/

Persaud, R. M.D. & Bruggen, P., M.D. (2012). *When Doctors Go On Strike Patients Stop Dying.* HuffPost Lifestyle. Retrieved from http://www.huffingtonpost.co.uk/dr-raj-persaud/when-doctors-go-on-strike_b_1513689.html

Reese, S. (2014). *Drug Abuse Among Doctors: Easy, Tempting, and Not Uncommon.* Medscape. Retrieved from http://www.medscape.com/viewarticle/819223

Riner, M., M.D. (2014). *Why patients have lost trust in their doctors.* Retrieved from http://www.kevinmd.com/blog/2014/02/patients-lost-trust-doctors.html

Starfield B., M.D. (2000). *Is US Health Really the Best in the World?* JAMA, 284(4):483-485. Retrieved from doi:10.1001/jama.284.4.483.

Chapter 10: An American Love Affair with Medications

Breakthrough Care Center. (2014). *Are Your Medicines Working Their Best for You?* Health and Wellness. Retrieved from http://breakthroughcarecenter.com/patient-resources/health-and-wellness/post/Are-Your-Medicines-Working-Their-Best-for-You

CDC. (2014). *Therapeutic Drug Use.* Retrieved from http://www.cdc.gov/nchs/fastats/drug-use-therapeutic.htm

CHPA. (2015). *Statistics on OTC Use.* Consumer Healthcare Products Association. Retrieved from http://www.chpa.org/marketstats.aspx

Gu, Q., M.D., Ph.D.; Dillon, C. F., M.D., Ph.D.; & Burt,V. L., Sc.M., R.N. (2010). *Prescription Drug Use Continues to Increase: U.S. Prescription Drug Data for 2007–2008.* Centers for Disease Control. Retrieved from http://www.cdc.gov/nchs/data/databriefs/db42.pdf

Huffington Post. (2013). *Serious, Sometimes Fatal Events May Occur: Why Do We Take So Many Drugs?* Retrieved from http://www.huffingtonpost.com/the-gypsynesters/prescription-drug-abuse-are-we-overmedicated_b_2464512.html

Kotz, D. (2010). *Overmedication: Are Americans Taking Too Many Drugs?* U.S. News & World Report. Health. Retrieved from http://health.usnews.com/health-news/managing-your-healthcare/diabetes/articles/2010/10/07/overmedication-are-americans-taking-too-many-drugs

Montgomery, J. (2014). *Prescription Drug Addiction.* HealthDay.com. Retrieved from http://consumer.healthday.com/encyclopedia/substance-abuse-38/drug-abuse-news-210/prescription-drug-addiction-648263.html

NIH. (2014). DrugFacts: *Prescription and Over-the-Counter Medications.* Retrieved from http://www.drugabuse.gov/publications/drugfacts/ prescription-over-counter-medications

Online-only: Prescription drug use on the rise in the United States. (2015). American Public Health Association. Retrieved from http://thenationshealth.aphapublications.org/content/40/8/ E37.full

Prescription Drug Abuse. (n.d.). Office of National Drug Control Policy. Retrieved from http://www.whitehouse.gov/ondcp/prescription-drug-abuse

Prime Therapeutics. (2014). Prime Therapeutics' Wickersham delivers keynote at Managed Markets Summit. Retrieved from http://www.primetherapeutics.com/Files/MMS_Keynote_ Press_Release_FINAL.pdf

Winstock. A. (2013). *Why America Has a Prescription Drug Epidemic: To Regulate Or Educate? No Question -- You Do Both.* Huffington Post. Retrieved from http://www. huffingtonpost.com/adam-winstock/why-america-has-a-prescri_b_4482058.html

Chapter 11: Let Food Be Your Medicine

Dehydrated products are healthy dog food alternatives. (2014). The Honest Kitchen. Retrieved from http://www.thehonestkitchen.com/why-choose-dehydrated-pet-food/

Guy, L. (2014). *Why eating makes you tired. Body & Soul.* Retrieved from http://www.bodyandsoul.com.au/nutrition/nutrition+tips/why+eating+makes+you+tired,9849

United States Department of Agriculture. (2011). Water in Meat and Poultry. Food Safety and Inspection Services. Retrieved from http://www.fsis.usda.gov/wps/wcm/connect/42a903e2-451d-40ea-897a-22dc74ef6e1c/Water_in_Meats.pdf?MOD=AJPERES

Chapter 12: Becoming Obese

Collins, S. P.K. (2014). *Fast Food Companies Keep Targeting Black Kids More Than Other Groups.* ThinkProgress.
Retrieved from http://thinkprogress.org/health/2014/11/13/3592198/fast-food-target-black-kids/

Cowling, L. L., M.P.H., R.D. (2006). *California Food Guide: Fulfilling the Dietary Guidelines for Americans.* Retrieved from http://www.dhcs.ca.gov/formsandpubs/publications/CaliforniaFoodGuide/17HealthandDietaryIssuesAffectingAfricanAmericans.pdf

Desmond-Harris, J. (2012). *On Blacks and Fat:* Chef Aaron McCargo Jr. Retrieved from http://www.theroot.com/articles/culture/2012/05/black_obesity_legacy_of_unhealthy_eating.html

Gaines, Dr. T. (2010). *How Obesity has become a part of black culture.* Retrieved from http://thegrio.com/2010/06/21/how-obesity-has-become-a-part-of-black-culture/

Heald, C. (2007). *Going ape.* BBC News, UK.
Retrieved from http://news.bbc.co.uk/2/hi/uk_news/magazine/6248975.stm

Kitahara, C.M., et al. (2014). *Association between Class III Obesity (BMI of 40–59 kg/m) and Mortality: A Pooled Analysis of 20 Prospective Studies.* PLOS Medicine, DOI: 10.1371/journal.pmed.1001673. Retrieved from http://www.nih.gov/news/health/jul2014/nci-08.htm

Laidman, J. (2013). *Obesity's Toll: 1 in 5 Deaths Linked to Excess Weight.* Medscape. Retrieved from http://www.medscape.com/viewarticle/809516#vp_2

McKenzie, B. (2010). *Raw Meat and Bone Diets for Dogs: It's Enough to Make You BARF. Science-Based Medicine.* Retrieved from http://www.sciencebasedmedicine.org/raw-meat-and-bone-diets-for-dogs-its-enough-to-make-you-barf/

Pitcairn R.H. & Pitcairn S.H. (2005). *Dr. Pitcairn's complete guide to natural health for dogs and cats,* 3rd ed. Rodale. As cited on http://www.sciencebasedmedicine.org/raw-meat-and-bone-diets-for-dogs-its-enough-to-make-you-barf/

Chapter 13: Reality Check—Exercise, Weight Loss, Obesity

Ajmera, R. (2013) *The Effects of Poor Nutrition on Your Health,* Livestrong. Retrieved from http://www.livestrong.com/article/31172-effects-poor-nutrition-health/

Allison, D.B. (2014) *Diet Myth: Eat Healthy Foods, and You'll Lose Weight.* Cooking Light. Retrieved from http://www.cookinglight.com/eating-smart/eat-healthy-foods-lose-weight-myth

Bailor, J. (2014) *The Calorie Myth: Why Eating Less & Exercising More Is NOT the Best Way to Burn Fat.* Retrieved from http://www.saragottfriedmd.com/the-calorie-myth-why-eating-less-exercising-more-is-not-the-best-way-to-burn-fat/

Best 10 Body Myths From Weigh Loss to Memory Loss, How Well Do You Know Your Body? (2006). 20/20, ABC News. Retrieved from http://abcnews.go.com/2020/story?id=2109291&page=1.

Bouchez, C. (2005-2014). *10 Diet Rules Meant to be Broken.* WebMD. Retrieved from http://www.webmd.com/diet/features/10-diet-rules-meant-to-be-broken

Comparison of vitamin levels in raw vs. cooked foods (2014). Beyond Vegetarianism. Retrieved from http://www.beyondveg.com/tu-j-l/raw-cooked/raw-cooked-2f.shtml

Familiarity With Television Fast-Food Ads Linked to Obesity. (2012). American Academy of Pediatrics. Retrieved from http://www.aap.org/en-us/about-the-aap/aap-press-room/Pages/Familiarity-With-Television-Fast-Food-Ads-Linked-to-Obesity.aspx

Gastric Bypass Surgery Gone Bad. Study: 1 in 50 People Die Within A Month of Surgery. (2005) CBS News. Retrieved from http://cbsnews.com/stories/2005/01/21/earlyshow/contributors/melindamurphy/main668323.shtml.

Greenfield, B. (2013). *Is "No Pain, No Gain" an Exercise Myth? Get-Fit Guy, Quick and Dirty Tips.* Retrieved from http://www.quickanddirtytips.com/health-fitness/exercise/is-%E2%80%9Cno-pain-no-gain%E2%80%9D-an-exercise-myth

Kolata, G. (2007). *Study Says Obesity Can Be Contagious,* Health. The New York Times. Retrieved from http://www.nytimes.com/2007/07/25/health/25cnd-fat.html?_r=0

Milken, M. (2008). *Choosing to Make America Healthie.,* San-Diego Tribune. Milken Institute. Retrieved from http://www.milkeninstitute.org/publications/view/348

Moss, Richard (2014). *Hereditary gut microbes found to influence weight gain.* Gizmag. Retrieved from http://www.gizmag.com/hereditary-gut-microbes-obesity/34661/

Obesity Surgeries Have Jumped Dramatically Since 1998. (2007). Agency for Healthcare Research and Quality. Retrieved from http://archive.ahrq.gov/news/press/pr2007/obesjumppr.htm

Sexton, T. (2011). *Does Food Lose Nutritional Value After Being Cooked?* Livestrong. Retrieved from http://www.livestrong.com/article/543167-does-food-lose-nutritional-value-after-being-cooked/

Shelley, J. (2012). *Addressing the policy cacophony does not require more evidence: an argument for reframing obesity as caloric overconsumption.* BioMed Central. Retrieved from http://www.biomedcentral.com/content/pdf/1471-2458-12-1042.pdf

Stoppler, M.C., M.D. & Shiel, Jr., W.C., M.D. (2014) *Stress, Hormones, and Weight Gain.* MedicineNet.com. Retrieved from http://www.medicinenet.com/script/main/art.asp?articlekey=53304

Warren-Gash, C. (2014) *Gut bacteria contributing to weight gain may be inherited.* BioNews. Retrieved from http://www.bionews.org.uk/page_468041.asp

Chapter 14: Coronary Heart Disease

Chelation: Therapy or "Therapy"? (2010). National Capital Poison Center. Retrieved from http://www.poison.org/current/chelationtherapy.htm

Link Between Cholesterol And Heart Disease Explained. (2007). Saint Louis University. ScienceDaily. Retrieved from www.sciencedaily.com/releases/2007/09/ 070918100608.htm.

Chapter 15: Plantarian Lifestyle for the Family

Body Image. (2014). Opposing Viewpoints in Context. Gale Cengage Learning. Retrieved from http://ic.galegroup.com/ic/ovic/Reference DetailsPage/DocumentToolsPortletWindow? displayGroupName=Reference&jsid=985b101159a45190b91a569c26ccd971&action=2&catId =GALE%7C00000000LVVJ &documentId=GALE%7CPC3010999221&u=cant48040&zid=4c5e0fd2f6e3d1e21c4aa1cfb88cdddc

Chapman, K. (2014). *Will a vegetarian diet reduce your risk of cancer?* Retrieved from http://www.abc.net.au/health/talkinghealth/factbuster/stories/ 2014/03/13/3962359.htm

Chronic Kidney Disease: Nutritional Considerations. (n.d.). Nutrition MD. Retrieved from http://www.nutritionmd.org/health_care_providers/renal/kidney_nutrition.html

Craig, W.J. & Mangels, A.R. (2009). (Abstract). *Position of the American Dietetic Association: vegetarian diets.* American Dietetic Association. Retrieved from http://www.ncbi.nlm.nih.gov/pubmed/19562864

Deans, B. (2008). *Many aging boomers who turned on in '60s stay addicted.* Orlando Sentinel. Cox News Service. Retrieved from http://articles.orlandosentinel.com/ 2008-09-05/news/drugs05_1_substance-abuse-substance-abuse-survey-on-drug

Gillman M.W. (2008). *The first months of life: a critical period for development of obesity.* American Journal of Clinical Nutrition, 87(6), 1587-9.

King, D., MS, RD. (2014). *Does eating a vegetarian diet help you live longer?* Vegetarian Nutrition. Retrieved from http://vegetariannutrition.net/vegetarian-diets/does-eating-a-vegetarian-diet-help-you-live-longer/

Kral, T.V. E., PhD & Faith, M.S., PhD (2009). *Influences on Child Eating and Weight Development From a Behavioral Genetics Perspective.* Journal of Pediatric Psychology. Retrieved from http://www.medscape.com/viewarticle/710209_6

McDougall, J.A. (2014). *Hormone Dependent Diseases (Male & Female).* Dr. McDougall's Health & Medical Center. Retrieved from https://www.drmcdougall.com/ health/education/health-science/common-health-problems/hormone-dependent-diseases-male-female/

Problem of Childhood Obesity Within a Generation. (2010). White House Task Force on Childhood Obesity Report to the President. Retrieved from http://www.letsmove.gov/ sites/letsmove. gov/files/TaskForce_on_Childhood_Obesity_May2010_FullReport.pdf

Vegetarian Diets in Chronic Kidney Disease. (2010). Academy of Nutrition and Dietetics. Retrieved from http://vegetariannutrition.net/docs/Renal-Vegetarian-Nutrition.pdf

Vegetarian Foods: Powerful for Health. (n.d.). The Physicians Committee For Responsible Medicine. Retrieved from http://www.pcrm.org/pdfs/ health/infovegfoods.pdf

Chapter 16: Plant-Based Nutrition for Seniors

Bollinger, L. (2012). *Easy Ways to Eat 5 Fruits & Veggies Each Day*. SparkPeople. Retrieved from http://www.sparkpeople.com/resource/nutrition_articles.asp?id=161

Gates, D. (2014). *About the Body Ecology Diet.* Retrieved from http://bodyecology.com/aboutbed.php

Hardy, L.H., M.D. (1999-2003). *How to free your body of toxins.* Global Institute for Alternative Medicine. Retrieved from http://www.med.nyu.edu/crs/assets/alternativemedicine.pdf

Huff, E.A. (2013). *Six amazing foods for cleansing your colon naturally.* Natural News. Retrieved from http://www.naturalnews.com/038680_ coloncleansing_ foods_apple_ cider_vinegar.html

Masterson, L., M.D. (2013). *Don't be afraid to speak honestly with your doctor.* SunSentinel. Retrieved from http://articles.sun-sentinel.com/2013-06-11/health/fl-jjps-doctor-0612-20130611_1_doctor-health-many-questions

Richmond, C. (2014). *23 Ways to Eat Clean. Prevention.* Retrieved from http://www.prevention.com/food/healthy-eating-tips/23-ways-eat-clean

Not Nice To Fool Mother Nature Commercial. (Uploaded 2010) Blast from the Past. Retrieved from https://www.youtube.com/watch?v=9q6QkUaXx_A

Chapter 17: Energy—How to "Bottle It!"

Ask.com (2014). *How do humans get energy?* Retrieved from http://www.ask.com/health/humans-energy-14ea640dbf74095c

Breus, M.J., PhD. (2013). *Sleep Newzzz: Sleep and diet have a powerful effect on each other.* Psychology Today. Retrieved from http://www.psychologytoday.com/blog/sleep-newzzz/201303/less-sleep-means-more-calories

Fight Stress With Food? Yes, Really! (2014). Today's Dietitian Health & Nutrition Center. Retrieved from http://www.todaysdietitian.com/ healthandnutrition/health/ fight-stress-with-food.shtml

Glassman, K., MS, RD, CDN. (2014). *13 Foods That Fight Stress.* Prevention. Retrieved from http://www.prevention.com/mind-body/emotional-health/13-healthy-foods-reduce-stress-and-depression

Mantica, A. (2014). *Sleep Well: What to Eat for Better Sleep.* Fitness Magazine. Retrieved from http://www.fitnessmagazine.com/health/sleep/what-to-eat-for-better-sleep/

Orenstein, B.W. (2014). *9 Foods That Help or Hurt Anxiety.* Anxiety Disorders. Everyday Health. Retrieved from http://www.everydayhealth.com/anxiety-pictures/anxiety-foods-that-help-foods-that-hurt-0118.aspx#03

Shaw, J. (2010). *Anti-Anxiety Foods and Vitamins.* LiveStrong.com. Retrieved from http://www.livestrong.com/article/311645-anti-anxiety-foods-and-vitamins/

WebMD (2014). *Chronic Pain Management.* Pain Management Health Center. Retrieved from http://www.webmd.com/pain-management/guide/understanding-pain-management-chronic-pain

Chapter 18: The Supplement Scam

Abse, N. (2012). *Nutrition, the new (old) way: Eat your vitamins—don't pop them.* Federal Soup. Retrieved from http://federalsoup.com/articles/2012/04/18/hf-story-1-nutrition-the-new-way--eat-your-vitamins-don-t-pop-them.aspx

Bakalar, N. (2013). *Dangers of Too Much Calcium.* The New York Times. Retrieved from http://well.blogs.nytimes.com/2013/02/18/dangers-of-too-much-calcium/?_r=0

Brody, J. (1995). *Study Links Excess Vitamin A and Birth Defects.* The New York Times. Retrieved from http://www.nytimes.com/1995/10/07/us/study-links-excess-vitamin-a-and-birth-defects.html

Dietary Supplements: What You Need to Know. (2014). Food Facts. U.S. Food & Drug Administration. Retrieved from http://www.fda.gov/Food/ResourcesForYou/Consumers/ ucm109760.htm

Dwyer, L. (2014). *Breakfast Bombshell: Vitamin Overload in Cereals May Be Making Kids Sick.* Takepart. Retrieved from http://www.takepart.com/article/2014/06/24/another-reason-worry-about-that-box-breakfast-cereal

Feskanich, D., Singh, V., Willett, W.C. & Colditz G.A. (2002). *Vitamin A Intake and Hip Fractures Among Postmenopausal Women.* JAMA, 2002;287(1):47-54. Retrieved from http://jama.jamanetwork.com/article. aspx?articleid=194525

Finz, S. (2004). SAN ANSELMO / *PowerBar founder collapses, dies at 51 / Athlete built empire on sports nutrition.* SF Gate. Retrieved from http://www.sfgate.com/bayarea/article/SAN-ANSELMO-PowerBar-founder-collapses-dies-at-2778452.php

Gann, C. (2011). *Women Taking Diet Supplements Should Think Twice, Study Says.* ABC News. Retrieved from http://abcnews.go.com/Health/vitamin-mineral-diet-supplements-harm-older-women-study/story?id=14706684

Goodman, B. (2014). *Healthy Adults Shouldn't Take Vitamin E, Beta Carotene: Expert Panel.* HealthDay. Retrieved from http://consumer.healthday.com/vitamins-and-nutrition-information-27/beta-carotene-news-57/healthy-adults-should-not-take-vitamin-e-beta-carotene-expert-panel-685178.html

Offit, P. (2013). *The Vitamin Myth: Why We Think We Need Supplements.* The Atlantic. Retrieved from http://www.theatlantic.com/health/ archive/2013/07/the-vitamin-myth-why-we-think-we-need-supplements/277947/

Schmidt, C. (2014). *Does cereal have too many vitamins for kids?* CNN Health. Retrieved from http://www.cnn.com/2014/06/25/health/cereal-vitamins-kids/

Chapter 19: The Perils of Physical Fitness

Cuomo, C. (2006). *Gym Germs Can Make You Sick.* ABC News. Retrieved from http://abcnews.go.com/gma/oncall/story?id=2237306

Galbraith, M. (2014). *How To Tell If Your Trainer Knows What They're Doing.* Retrieved from http://mollygalbraith.com/2012/02/how-to-tell-if-your-trainer-knows-what-theyre-doing/

Goldhammer, K.A., Dooley, D.P., Avala, E., Zera, W., & Hill, B.L. (2006). *Prospective study of bacterial and viral contamination of exercise equipment.* US National Library of Medicine. National Institutes of Health. Retrieved from http://www.ncbi.nlm.nih.gov/pubmed/16377973

Jio, S. (2012). *Is Going to the Gym Making You ... Sick? New Report on Germs at the Gym.* Glamour.com. Retrieved from http://www.glamour.com/health-fitness/blogs/vitamin-g/2012/12/is-going-to-the-gym-making-you

Reyes, M. (2012). *Germs at the Gym.* Fitness Magazine. Retrieved from http://www.fitnessmagazine.com/health/germs/germs-at-the-gym/

Rodrigues, A. (2014). *I Went To A Personal Trainer (So You Don't Have To) And It Was Totally Weird.* Thought Catalogue. Retrieved from http://thoughtcatalog.com/ashwin-rodrigues/2014/03/i-went-to-a-personal-trainer-so-you-dont-have-to-and-it-was-totally-weird/

Schwecherl, L. (2011). *Are Germs at the Gym Making You Sick?* Greatest.com. Retrieved from http://greatist.com/fitness/are-germs-gym-making-you-sick

Wilson, J. (2014). *Investigation: The Ten Filthiest Objects at the Gym (With Germs That Can Make You Sick!).* A Natural News Investigation. Retrieved from http://www.naturalnews.com/filthiest-objects-gym-germs.html

Wooldridge, L.Q. (2012). *Don't Get Sick at the Gym: 7 Ways to Prevent Infection.* Health. US News. Retrieved from http://health.usnews.com/health-news/articles/2012/04/25/dont-get-sick-at-the-gym-7-ways-to-prevent-infection

Chapter 20: "Trish's Story"

Body Ecology. (2006). *How to Eat Your Vegetables Raw (With NO Gas or Bloating!).* Retrieved from http://bodyecology.com/articles/raw_vegetables_gas_bloating.php#.VKQzTdLF8YE

Godwin, C. (2013). *How to Reduce Swelling With These Fruits.* LiveStrong. Retrieved from http://www.livestrong.com/article/530975-how-to-reduce-swelling-with-these-fruits/

Hill, S.C. (2013). *Obesity and Skin Care Management.* LivesStrong.com. Retrieved from http://www.livestrong.com/article/75355-obesity-skin-care-management/

Loomis, H.F., D.C. (2014). *Autointoxication.* Loomis Institute. Retrieved from http://www.loomisinstitute.com/articles/autointoxication.aspx?list=bydate

Rose, D. (2013). *Too Many Vegetables? How To Prevent Gas and Digestive Problems Caused By Healthy Eating.* Retrieved from http://summertomato.com/too-many-vegetables-how-to-prevent-gas-and-digestive-problems-caused-by-healthy-eating/

SparkPeople. (2014). *Nutrition Facts: Calories in taco bell nacho bell grande.* Retrieved from http://www.sparkpeople.com/calories-in.asp?food=taco+bell+nacho+bell+grande

Wakamatsu, M., M.D. (2010-2014). *How does obesity contribute to urinary incontinence?* ShareCare. Retrieved from http://www.sharecare.com/health/urinary-incontinence/obesity-contribute-to-urinary-incontinence

Chapter 21: What Goes In Must Come Out

Carrera, A.L. (n.d.). *The Best Foods to Eat for Healthy Bowel Movements.* SFGate. Retrieved from http://healthyeating.sfgate.com/foods-eat-healthy-bowel-movements-1754.html

Jaimison, M. (2013). *Can Constipation Cause Heart Attacks?* ACLS.com. Retrieved from http://www.aclscertification.com/blog/can-constipation-cause-heart-attacks/

Roizman, T. (2014). *Will Eating Lots of Fruit and Vegetables Cleanse Your System?* Demand Media. Retrieved from http://healthyeating.sfgate.com/eating-lots-fruit-vegetables-cleanse-system-8942.html

WiseGeek. (2003-2014). *What Are the Symptoms of Vagus Nerve Damage?* WiseGeek.com. Retrieved from http://www.wisegeek.org/what-are-the-symptoms-of-vagus-nerve-damage.htm

Chapter 22: Shopping for Plantarian Foods

American RadioWorks (2015). *GM Crops: The Arguments Pro and Con.* Retrieved from http://americanradioworks.publicradio.org/features/gmos_india/pro_con2.html

Colbert, T. (2014). *GMOs: Pros and Cons.* Healthline.com. Retrieved from http://www.healthline.com/health/gmos-pros-and-cons

Colby, M. (2014). *Nuclear Lunch: The Dangers of Radiation-Exposed Foods.* Retrieved from http://www.foodandwater.org/?page_id=8

Duvauchelle, J. (2014). *Pros & Cons of GMO Foods.* LiveStrong.com. Retrieved from http://www.livestrong.com/article/213053-pros-cons-of-gmo-foods/

Institute for Responsible Technology. (2006-2014). *10 Reasons to Avoid GMOs.* Retrieved from http://www.responsibletechnology.org/10-Reasons-to-Avoid-GMOs

Lippert, M. (2015). *Q. Organic—or Not? Is Organic Produce Healthier Than Conventional?* Eating Well. Retrieved from http://www.eatingwell.com/food_news_origins/green_sustainable/organic_or_not_is_organic_ produce_healthier_than_conventional

The Decuypere Report. (2014). *Genetically Engineered Foods.* Retrieved from http://www.health-alternatives.com/ge-foods-report.html

Walia, A. (2014). *10 Scientific Studies Proving GMOs Can Be Harmful To Human Health.* Retrieved from http://www.collective-evolution.com/2014/04/08/10-scientific-studies-proving-gmos-can-be-harmful-to-human-health/

Watson, S. (2012). *Organic food no more nutritious than conventionally grown food. Harvard Health Publications.* Harvard Medical School. Retrieved from http://www.health.harvard.edu/blog/organic-food-no-more-nutritious-than-conventionally-grown-food-201209055264

Webber, V. (2014) *22 Pros and Cons Organic and Conventional Agriculture.* Retrieved from http://www.slideboom.com/presentations/32462/22Pros-and-Cons-organic-and-conventional-agriculture%5B1%5D

Whole Foods. (2014). *Is Organic Food Better For You?* Retrieved from http://www.wholefoodsmarket.com/mission-values/organic/organic-food-better-you

www.ingramcontent.com/pod-product-compliance
Lightning Source LLC
LaVergne TN
LVHW091046080826
845145LV00002B/644

* 9 7 8 0 9 8 3 7 2 2 9 6 0 *